The Looking Mask

A Journey Through Cancer

Also by Stephen Krueger

Island of the Son

Ten Thousand and a Wake-Up

Stephen

Krueger

ISBN: 0692560823
ISBN-13:9780692560822

DEDICATION

To my wife Susan and my family.

To the doctors, nurses, technicians and everyone involved in fighting cancer for us all.

To Professor Marie Hara, for your encouragement and belief in me.

CONTENTS

CONTENTS

THE LOOKING MASK

A JOURNEY THROUGH CANCER

PROLOGUE

I AM STILL HERE. Over three years later and I am still here. Every day it gets a little easier for me, but every day, without exception, I think about it and know that it can devastate, or even end my life. Some days are harder than others. Some days, like today, I struggle with the loss of people I don't even know. I spend more time thinking about it than anything else in my life. Every day I pray it won't come back.

I don't know how it happened to me. I still struggle to understand how it happened. It can happen to anyone. Don't think it can't. One day your life is idling along and the next day it turns on its head.

My life will never be the same as it was. It will always be different. Once upon a time, I thought I was indestructible. It could happen to other people but not to me. I thought I was in control of my life. I did most of the right things to prevent it, but that wasn't enough, it came and got me anyway. It came and got me from long ago. It's a remnant of a time and place that I haven't seen for thirty-eight years.

This is the story of what happened to my body and mind. Physically some of the effects are still there. I am told some things will never be the same as they once were, but the physical leftovers are nothing compared to what happened to me mentally.

Outside my family, of which there are few, and my doctors/nurses (probably most of whom don't remember me) maybe ten people know.

In many ways it has wrecked me. I'm so afraid that if I talk about it with others it will come back stronger and punish me worse. I'm petrified that I'm the mole in the *Whack a Mole* game.

When I do talk about it, I am always on the verge of collapse. You probably wouldn't know - but I do.

By the grace of God, my family, my doctors, my nurses and countless others I AM STILL HERE. Maybe I shouldn't put that in CAPS.

Here goes.

I HAD CANCER

I hope this story helps.

Day 1 – Tuesday - May 31, 2011

Today is my first day of radiation treatments and my first chemotherapy session. It's a twofer. I am terrified. I have been hiding from it the last week, trying to cover it up and bury my head in the sand like this day was never coming. Nothing works. I can't spend a minute not thinking about it. I dream about it. I wake-up over and over and the first thing I do is think about it.

Last weekend my wife Susan and I went to the Oregon Coast. If anything would take me away from my thoughts, it would be the water but even that didn't work. I tried to meditate but my head won't clear. My brain is a record needle stuck in a groove.

I think about the malformed deadly cells that are most likely multiplying inside of me incessantly. I considered not showing up today. Dr. Lee said that my cancer was gone from what they could tell, but he also said it would almost definitely come back without radiation and chemotherapy. Quite a choice, do something where they tried to almost kill you or do nothing and it would probably kill you. Almost or probably, it was up to me. In the end, I went with almost, hoping they wouldn't overshoot their goal.

This morning, I put myself in a self-induced daze, probably from the lack of sleep and nerves, and went through the motions. We drove to the Willamette Valley Cancer Institute, parked, checked in and paid twenty-four dollars for the day's treatment. I gave Susan a perfunctory kiss, dropped her off in the waiting room, went to the patient locker room, took off my shirt, put on a silly medical frock and stepped into the small waiting room where I joined four or five women, no men, and waited for my name to be called.

As soon as I sat down, I grabbed a magazine from a cheap faux wood side table. I don't know what magazine it was and I certainly didn't read it. I didn't even look at the pictures, I just picked it up so I could avoid talking to anyone in the room.

I sat there in dismay, wondering how I could end up at a cancer institute. I'm in my early fifties, been married to the same woman for thirty-four years, have three children ages thirty-four, thirty-one and twenty-one, and three grandsons. I grew up in Wisconsin and Belize and joined the Navy at the age of eighteen. Went from Seaman Recruit to Commander during my almost twenty-eight years in the Navy. Started washing dishes and ended up leading hundreds of young men and women. The only time I ever missed a day of work for sickness was when I had pneumonia and they put me in the hospital for a couple of days, and the day they had me swallow Iodine 131 for Graves' disease. How the hell did I end up here? What did I do to deserve this?

I'm not sure how long it was, maybe five or ten minutes, before a technician came to the entrance of the cubicle and called my name.

Everything went according to plan, my panic and fear outwardly under control, until I neared the entrance to the room where the machine was housed.

"Okay Steve, right in here," the no name, blurred face specialist said. He motioned me closer to the door.

I stepped forward, he opened the door and I entered. I took one step into the room and stopped cold. The machine that would possibly save my life sat there without expression, staring at me, not making a sound. :::::Please God, help me.::::: It sat about twenty feet away and was at least twelve feet long and ten feet wide at its far end. Portions of it must have been nine feet tall. Closest to me was a metal slab which was about eight feet long with holes for bolts along the sides. The slab, with me attached to it, would slide into what looked like a donut in the middle of the machine. The donut, itself contained within the larger machine, would spin around me and precisely shoot radiation into my head and neck region to hopefully rid me of the cancer in my body. :::::Hopefully, hopefully.::::: If there was any.

The machine and I stared at each other for a few unmoving seconds. I blinked first and slowly walked forward to meet my new best friend. This piece of metal and plastic and fiberglass and circuits and glass and lights, as directed by technicians and doctors and nurses and researchers, which were directed by a higher power would do one of three things. It would get it right, get it wrong and not remove all the cancer, or kill me.

Eventually I made it to the metal slab and stopped once again. "Okay, please lie down, just like we practiced last week," the technician said as he walked over to a set of lockers on the left side of the room. I sat down on the freezing shiny slab and watched him go to a locker which had a piece of tape with my name written in crayon or magic marker or whatever writing instrument they used to designate lockers for the temporary storage of gear for us temporary patients. Nobody was permanent here. He opened the door of the locker, reached in and *presto* out came a hardened mesh mold of my head and shoulders. "Looks just like you," he said looking at the mold and back at me. "Lie down and relax."

:::::Are you kidding me? You f'in relax!::::: I so much wanted to say, but I restrained myself knowing he was doing his best to make me comfortable. Relaxing was a lost cause today, it didn't matter what he did or what he said or how many times we practiced, I was not going to "relax."

Without saying a word, I slowly lay down. The cold medical steel shocked me through the medical frock which only partially covered my back. I turned my head to the right to look at him as he approached me with that mold.

:::::Get up and run. Run now, you can make it. They cannot make you do this.::::: As he arrived, I turned my head front and center and he brought the hardened restraint over my face and shoulders. In a couple of seconds I would be completely immobile from my shoulders on up. :::::Run, Run.:::::

"Okay, slide forward a little," he said.

I sucked it up and did as he requested. The mold finished its trek and covered my upper torso perfectly. "You're doing great," he said.

I heard him grab bolts and fasteners from his pocket.

:::::Last chance, sit up and run.::::: A bolt slid through a hole in the medal slab and he screwed the fastener on. :::::Too late.:::::

He fastened the remaining bolts. By the time the sixth bolt was secured I could hardly breathe. I'm not sure if it was from the panic or the tightness of the mask. Maybe a combination of both.

"Perfect," he said. "Are you okay?"

"I'm fine," I said, my lips brushing the mesh as I talked. :::::I am not okay, I have cancer. Hurry up, get out of this room and turn the damn machine on. Let it do its thing before I scream. Get me out of this sterile damn building, where people are dying and everyone is masquerading, pretending everything is going to be just fine.:::::

"Okay, Mr. Wendt, I'm going to the other room. This will take about fifteen minutes. Unlike when we practiced and didn't actually turn the machine on, this time you will hear and see the machine moving over you and spinning around. The machine will make clicking and clacking noises and lights will blink on and off. That's what it is supposed to do. Hang in there; I'll be back in no time. Do you want to listen to any music? There is a radio in here if you want to."

:::::Sure, could you release me from this trap and let me find a station I like, please?::::: "No, I'm good. Do what you have to do." :::::Just do it quickly please. No damn radio or music is going to make it better.:::::

I closed my eyes and a few seconds later the machine began to hum and move. At its first sound, I opened my eyes but closed them again as soon as I saw a red light flashing. I began to count. One thousand one, one thousand two, one thousand three. Fifteen minutes, that was only nine hundred seconds. One thousand four, one thousand five. That's not so long. One thousand six, that's forever, one thousand seven, one thousand eight, keep counting, one thousand nine, you are one percent done, only eight hundred and ninety seconds to go.

One thousand twenty……. Imagine what your father went through. I should have been a better son. He was all alone, him and his damn leukemia, in a sterile room with a window, where once in a while they dripped poison into him and called it chemotherapy. How he must have longed to leave that room when he looked out that fifth floor, cancer ward, sterile room window at the people below. How he must have prayed that by some miracle he would get better when he stared at the cream colored walls, alone, yet surrounded by five billion people outside that little ten by twelve, germ free space.

Here I was, all alone. Me, my mask and my machine. Unable to move for the next fourteen minutes and thirty seconds before I could run away from this personal jail. Fifteen minutes, big deal. Imagine how my father had to do it, twenty-four hours a day, 1440 minutes a day, 86,400 seconds. :::::Try counting that out to get away from what's happening to you dummy. And then when you are done counting, do it over and over again, day after day. Be grateful it's only nine hundred seconds.:::::

I could have done so much better for my father. He went through chemotherapy - twice. The first time he was locked down for about thirty days before they set him free and the second time around, about a year after the first, it killed him. The second time he went into that room, he never left.

In the end, he was alone in that sterile room, facing the fact that he was probably going to die there and I called him once every other day from work in Hawai'i. I know he looked forward to those calls. He never let me know that he needed me more and always seemed grateful for the calls. I thought he would walk out of that room again. He did not. I wish now that I had called him every day. Every single day, twice a day. I wish I had gone to visit him earlier instead of arriving one day before he died. You knew it was bad when they let everyone in his sterile room that last day. I guess it didn't matter at that point and he started to fade in and out two or three hours after I arrived.

Up until that last day, I was so consumed in myself, my job, and my family, sadly in that order, that I thought there would be time. There was not. The amount of time he had was not up to me. Why, why, why didn't I do better? I should have done more. Why?

He was my first memory even though he was my adopted father. I remember being in a crib, I don't know, maybe I was a year and one-half or two years old. I remember looking up and seeing his younger self, jet black semi-curly hair, brown eyes and ruddy face. He was looking down at me with a smile. My mother, my grandfather and my grandmother were in that memory as well, but they were not the focus. He was the focus. I think it was the only thing I remembered before the age of five and his image has always stayed with me. Even now I, over fifty years later, can call up that memory whenever I want it.

He was a good man. I'm sure he always tried his best. Don't we all? He was by no means perfect and he and I had huge differences, but I am forever indebted to him. He didn't owe me a thing. Nothing. What he did for me couldn't be measured. He sacrificed for me when he had no obligation to do so.

I found out at the age of thirteen that I was his adopted son. Prior to that I had no idea. None. It came out after he and I had our first fight. That fight was the first time that I stood up to him. I don't even remember what it was about. I think he told me to do something and I told him he couldn't make me. In the early seventies, in our house, that behavior was not tolerated. I'm sure I took a spanking with the dog leash and did what I was told to do in the end, but the bigger shock came the next day. I will always remember my mother sitting me down and saying, "Your father is not your father. I am your mother but he is not your father." My dumb response was asking her, "How old am I?" Really? "How old am I?" What did that have to do with anything? Oh well, I was in shock. I wish I had asked any other question but that stupid one, but that was the one I asked.

To this day I have not asked the question of who my "real" father was. Whenever it enters my head for a second, I dismiss it. Gunthar Wendt was my real father. When he married my mother, after he had already been through so much during his life, including a war where he was bombed every night, in the "old country," he became my father. From my perspective he never treated me any different than my brother or sister. He was hard, very hard. By today's standards his actions would probably be called abuse, but I never thought of it that way.

My real father was not the bum who I shared my DNA with and who I probably looked exactly like. My real father was not the bum who knocked up my mother in 1957 and never wrote or called me. The guy who gave me his DNA was just a sperm donor. That's right - I am pissed at you. How could you? I've never met you, but the way you treated me has had a huge impact on what I am today, both good and bad. I never feel as if I am good enough. That is on me, but it's also on you, whoever you are.

For the last ten years of his life, I knew if I needed to I could have called my true father, Gunthar Wendt, anytime and he would have done his best to be there. I wish I could call him now, but that boat sailed in October 2001 when he died from the disease in which his cells were taken over and destroyed in that sterile damn room receiving chemotherapy treatments which went past the "almost" line.

He died all alone, since we had all gone to the hotel for the evening thinking he would make it until tomorrow. But he had no more tomorrows. I got a call an hour after I checked into the hotel and was told that he had died. An hour after he died I was in the hospital again.

I sat with him there in that sterile room, just he and I. The machines were all off, no more IV bags, no more chemo, no more lines running into him, no more grandchildren, no more talking on the phone, no more anything in this life for him. He looked young to me again, like the man I saw when I was a baby, not the sixty-nine year old man I had seen earlier in the day, fading in and out under the control of ever increasing dosages of morphine.

:::::Please Lord, take care of my father. Please take him to heaven to be with you. Please.:::::

I sat with his body for about fifteen minutes before a nurse came in.

"He knew this therapy probably wouldn't work but he did this experimental chemotherapy anyway, hoping he would help others in the future."

Gunthar Wendt was my father, I wish I had been a better son. I could have done so much more, so much. Why did I waste all that time? I wish I had….

"Okay Steve," a voice said. My brain jerked and brought me back to reality. My head would have jerked along with my brain but it couldn't move a millimeter. "Let me loosen these bolts and you are done here for the day. I think you are going up to chemotherapy next. Nice job."

He unbolted me and I bolted upright. "Thanks, that wasn't so bad," I said. :::::Liar.:::::

I couldn't get off of that machine and out of that room fast enough. I headed to the patient locker room. Once there, I sat down in front of my locker and sighed. One down, thirty-four to go and all I had next was my first chemotherapy, just another four or five hour deal which I did not want to face. I slowly changed back into my shirt and put the gown into my locker. Another locker with my name written on tape for easy removal. I wondered how many others had put their gowns in that temporary locker and how many were still with us. :::::I hope it was a lucky locker, as if there is any such thing. I'll take it if there is.:::::

I exited the locker room and went to the waiting room where Susan was. I sat beside her.

"How did it go?" she asked.

"Just great," I said sarcastically. "Just like we practiced the other day, only completely different. They strapped me down and the machine spun around making all kinds of noises for the whole fifteen minutes. Plus this time it fired real bullets. No more blanks. I guess we can go to chemotherapy now. I am so looking forward to that. I just want to go home and forget about this."

"You know what the doctor said." She smiled at me, always encouraging. "You can handle this."

"Yeah, I can handle it." I got up, as did Sue, and we walked over and entered the elevator which would carry us to the tippy-top of the two-story Willamette Valley Cancer Institute. An elevator for a two story building? This place really was for people who were not feeling well. I wanted to walk up but I couldn't find the stairs.

A couple of seconds later we exited the elevator into the serene waiting room and reception area of the chemo floor. :::::How long could a two story elevator take?::::: No signs of anything medical in the waiting room and reception area other than a couple of placards. One pointed to a hallway which led to the Pharmacy and the other directed those inclined down a passageway to the Chemo Room. :::::That about covers it, they put this fake area out front for visitors and hid the sick people in the back.::::: We walked past the empty reception desk, through the empty chair filled room, and turned into the corridor which led to the Chemo Room. I must have been the last patient of the day, no other people were around. At the end of the corridor a door automatically opened and I was greeted by a friendly nurse.

"Stephen Wendt, correct?"

"Yes"

"Can I get your ID so we can verify we are giving this treatment to the right person?"

"Okay." I hesitated. "Do you really think somebody who didn't need this would volunteer to have chemotherapy? I kind of doubt it." :::::God knows that everyone wants some chemo. I know I wanted some before it was prescribed.::::: I pulled out my ID and handed it over.

"Just following procedures. You'd be surprised. Follow me," she said kindly. We walked over to a station with a large comfortable medical examining chair, a metal roller tray with medicine on it and a couple of waiting room chairs. The station was divided from other stations by a curtain which could wrap completely around the small area. "Sit down." She pointed to the medical examining chair which came complete with fold out arms, for easy access to my veins.

I sat and looked at the whole room. Around the perimeter of the large room were approximately fifteen set-ups just like mine. About ten of the stations were occupied. Almost all of the occupied stations had people sitting down, with IV bags slowly dripping into them. Many of the patients were bald or wearing hats or wraps around their heads. Some were skinny, some were pale, most were skinny and pale. Almost all were there with somebody. In the center of the room was a large rectangular nurse's station with three or four nurses milling about doing their thing.

"I'm Katherine," my nurse said. "Please get as comfortable as you can. We are going to do a large IV bag and a few smaller bags for you today."

I looked over and saw four bags, one large and three smaller ones sitting on the metal table.

"You don't have a central line, do you?" she asked.

"That's correct, I do not." I looked around the room again. Many of those at the stations had their bags hooked up into areas other than their arms. Central lines. Somebody, a doctor probably, mentioned me possibly getting a central line for my treatment, but I immediately rejected that idea. Why would I let them put a central line in me while I still had good veins in my arms? That meant you were really sick and I was not going there.

"Good, I'll stick you and then we can get the bags hooked up. See this slightly brown tinged solution?" she said holding it up. "That is 'The Magic'."

"Or 'The Killer,'" I said.

"The Magic," Susan said, looking me straight in my eyes.

Katherine put down "The Magic" and took a look at my left arm, where she saw the easily identifiable track marks of somebody who had been stuck about fifty times in the last two months and had given blood over the years. She grabbed a huge needle and I watched as she slipped that sharp piece of hallowed out metal into my arm like butter. I didn't even feel the penetration into my body. She taped the large needle onto my arm and quickly hooked me up to the large saline IV bag. "Just salt water," I thought, and then in a blink I watched her reach for the other smaller bags and she methodically hooked them to the drip. The last one she hooked up was "The Magic." Almost immediately, I saw it begin to dispense its poison into the line, one small brown drop at a time. When "The Magic" liquid intermixed with the remainder of the liquids which were all clear, it tinged the whole concoction to a khaki color. I looked down to where the line entered my arm and the brown liquid began to feed into me. This was the stuff that killed my father and my grandfather. I wanted to stand up, rip that needle out of my arm and scream "NO, NO, NO, I AM IN CHARGE OF THIS AND I SAY NO," but instead I sat there and watched the chemo bag drip ever so slowly, one drop every ten seconds or so. Into my arm it went, mixing with my blood, looking for the bad cells and hopefully destroying them if there were any. Nobody knew.

"Okay," Katherine said, "this is going to take three or four hours. I know you signed the forms concerning all the side effects previously. If you feel anything funny or different in any way, please let me know right away. The bathroom is right over there. You need to drink plenty of water. If you don't, the chemo can damage your kidneys and we don't want that. Also, when you are done I have a couple of prescriptions for nausea. The directions are on the bottles. You can take them as you need them. We'll go over that later."

"All right." My eyes were glued on the little brown bag dispensing poison into me.

"Are you okay? Look at me," Susan said. She tried to rip my stare from that bag, and check my level of fear.

Her words broke the spell the bag had over me but I averted her direct stare. I didn't want her to see my absolute terror, even though I knew she could read my fear without looking into my eyes. "I'm fine. Maybe I'll just try and sleep through this."

“Good luck with that. Let me know if you need anything. Water, food, whatever.”

“I will.” I closed my eyes and tried not to pay attention to what must have been a physical revolt inside me.

:::::How the hell did you end up here?:::::

It was 6:30 AM on Valentine’s Day 2011. I got up just like I always do, went to the bathroom, stood in front of the mirror and looked up. The left side of my neck was swollen. :::::What the heck was that?::::: There was a large bump, maybe two by two inches sticking out. I reached up and felt it. It felt like a lump of fat under my skin, maybe it was a swollen lymph node. I shrugged it off. It would go away. It was just a lump.

Happy Valentine’s Day.

It did not disappear.

March 7, 2011

“Do you have a cat?” Doctor Zurbringer asked without any inflection.

This guy sounded like a robot, how did I luck into this guy? “A cat? Yes we have a cat,” I replied.

“Has it ever scratched you?” He was feeling up the bumps on my neck.

“Not really, I suppose she could have, but I haven’t felt it.”

:::::You can squeeze the lumps all you want, they will still be there. Believe me, I know. I’ve squeezed them a thousand times.:::::

"These lumps on the side of your neck are pretty big. It seems you have two or three swollen lymph nodes and they can be caused by a cat scratch," he coldly stated.

"Like Cat Scratch Fever? Is that real?" I said. Come on doc, smile, make me feel a little better here.

His hands dropped from my neck but his look didn't change at all. Not even a make believe smile. "Yes. I am going to give you some antibiotics and see if that clears them up. If not, we'll try to figure out what else could be happening."

"Could it be something else?" I didn't like this at all.

"Maybe. Let's see what happens with this. If it doesn't clear up, come and see me in a couple of weeks."

"Should I worry?"

"It's up to you."

Wow, this guy had a real way with people. It was like talking to a droid.

I went home and took my pills.

March 21, 2011

Dr. Zurbringer was looking at me again, same expression – no expression. "It doesn't look like these have changed at all. I hoped the antibiotics would clear this up. We'll need to do some bloodwork. It could be serious."

"What does that mean?" I asked.

"We don't know yet. It could be anything. It could just be swollen lymph nodes which didn't respond to the antibiotics. We'll get some bloodwork and hopefully see what's going on. I'll let you know in a couple of days." He quietly stood and walked out of the examining room.

I guess he didn't want to talk any more. I had some questions, but apparently he didn't have any answers so he never got around to asking me if I had any questions. He dropped the word "serious" on me and then took off. This guy was perfect for a family practice doctor.

The nurse came in, took my blood and told me I could go home.

This clinic is so great. You sign in, they take your money and you are just another number to them. Nothing personal. Just business. Real nice. They make you feel like they really care.

March 28, 2011 – 11:30 AM

My cell phone rang. I pulled it out of my pocket and looked at the number. It was Dr. Zurbringer. I did not want to answer, but I did.

"Hello" :::::Please let it be nothing.:::::

He got right to it. "Mr. Wendt, this is Dr. Zurbringer. I have some news for you. We got the results of your bloodwork and you need to be prepared for the possibility that you have cancer."

"What?" I said. :::::Cancer? Where did that come from?:::::

"It looks like there is a very real possibility that you have cancer." Monotone the whole way.

I looked around. I was home alone. It was a typical Oregon day. It was wet, cold and just plain miserable. Nothing else to say about it. We had moved here from Hawai'i just a few months ago and I was not acclimated to the weather. Susan and our youngest daughter, Stacy, who was twenty-one, were out running errands. I sat down before I crumpled. "Cancer?"

"Yes," he replied. "I am going to schedule a scan of the swollen area and some other tests. You should be hearing from the people who perform the scan shortly. Do you have any other questions?"

I had a ton of questions, but I was in shock. I sat on the couch shaking my head. :::::Over the phone? Really? Over the phone? You tell me I might have cancer over the phone?:::::

"Mr. Wendt, are you there?"

:::::I should scream at you right now. You no-personality prick. I'm just another number to you, aren't I? If it weren't for the lumps on my neck, you wouldn't know me if I walked up to you and introduced myself. You are a real bedside manner guy. Thanks!:::: I shook my head. "Yes, I'm here." I rubbed my neck, the bumps were still there.

"As I said, you should be hearing from the scan people soon. Good-bye." He hung up.

I never heard from Dr. Zurbringer again. It was nice to be wanted. What a dick. You tell a man he probably has cancer over the phone and you never call him again. Honestly, I never wanted to talk to him again. The sooner I was rid of him the better. Clearly, he didn't give a damn about me.

Now what?

March 28, 2011 – 12:30 PM

"Mr. Wendt, this is the Ultrasound Clinic," a soothing voice said over the phone.

"Okay"

"Mr. Wendt, we have a priority request for a scan for you. Can you come in tomorrow?"

"What will you be doing?"

"Just a scan of the area that is swollen on your neck. It should only take about fifteen minutes. How about 1 PM tomorrow? We are only about fifteen minutes away from where you live."

"Okay, do I need to bring or do anything?" I rubbed the bumps on my neck while I was speaking. No matter how much I touched, rubbed, pushed or probed them they were always there.

"No, just bring yourself." She hung up.

March 28, 2011 - 2 PM

"Susan, I got a call today from the doctor about the lumps on my neck." I reached up and rubbed for about the millionth time.

"Stop rubbing them, it will make them bigger," she said.

"The doctor said I might have cancer."

"Cancer?"

"Yes, cancer."

"What did he say?"

"He called me and said that I need to be prepared for the 'very real possibility' that I have cancer and that I need some further tests. I am scheduled for an ultrasound of my neck tomorrow. This scares the hell out of me. What if I have cancer? We just retired and moved here and now I am told that I might have cancer?"

"You'll be fine, you don't have cancer."

"What if I do?" I reached up, but before I touched my neck I brought my hands down to my side.

"Then we will deal with it and get through it." She sighed. "Did he say what type of cancer?"

"No, just that there was a VERY REAL POSSIBILTY that I have cancer. He didn't say what type. I assume it has something to do with the lumps on my neck. I don't understand it. One day they just popped up, they don't hurt, they look worse than they feel. First he says maybe Cat

Scratch Fever and then we go to the real possibility that I have cancer. This is so screwed up. Maybe tomorrow I can find out."

"Don't assume you have cancer, we aren't there yet. Give me a hug please."

We stood and gave each other a hug. "That's enough, you can let me go now. You are squeezing a little too hard," Susan said.

I didn't want to let go. This can't be happening. Cancer?

March 29, 2011 - 1:14 PM

"Okay Mr. Wendt, just lie down on the table and we are going to smear some jelly on your neck. Do you want it warmed up or cold?"

"Whatever way is easiest for you. Is this just like a pregnancy ultrasound?"

"Yep, just like a pregnancy ultrasound. After we get some jelly on you, we are going to take the wand and rub it around the swollen area."

She smeared the warmed up stuff on my neck and proceeded to glide the wand over the bumps. It didn't take long.

"Okay Mr. Wendt, we're done, you can put your shirt back on and somebody will call you with the results in a day or so."

"Anything preliminary?" I asked.

"I'm not a doctor, so I don't know. The professionals will read it out and let you know the results."

"Come on now, I know you guys in the trenches know what's really going on. What do you think?"

"I really, really don't know," she said. "Really"

The more she said "really," the less I believed her. :::::Really?::::: "Come on, you can tell me," I said. "Please."

"I really, really, really don't know but if I were you I would go home and get drunk tonight."

"What does that mean? Is it that bad that I should go and get drunk?" I said.

"My comment meant nothing. I told you I don't know and I mean it. I wish I did know and could tell you, so you could feel better or know what was going on. Obviously you are pretty stressed out. I thought maybe a drink or two would help. I can't tell you anything. We'll get the results to you soon."

:::::Damn, Steve. She knows and it's not good.:::::

March 30, 2011 – 8 AM

"Mr. Wendt, this is the Oregon Medical Group Ear, Nose and Throat Clinic. Can you come in for an appointment to see Dr. Lee?"

"Why am I being seen by an Ear, Nose and Throat Doctor?" I asked.

"We received a call from your doctor, Doctor Zurbringer, and he said that after reviewing your ultrasound we need to get an appointment for you as soon as possible. Did he call you?"

"He did not." :::::Surprise, he didn't call me and let me know. Let somebody else do his dirty work. The sooner I was out of his hair the better for him.::::: "When is the appointment for?"

"How about today at 2 PM?"

"Okay, but why am I seeing an Ear, Nose and Throat Doctor?"

"As I said, you were referred to us, so we need to get you an appointment soonest. You can call your other doctor if you want. I am going to schedule you with Doctor Lee for 2 PM today. Is that okay? We are located in Eugene on Martin Luther King Boulevard. Please be here fifteen minutes ahead of time so you can check in."

"Okay, I'll be there." :::::Damn, that was quick. Same day service from a doctor. That ultrasound was so bad that I need to be seen today. How serious was this? These lumps must be something bad, but why an Ear, Nose and Throat guy? Is there something I can't see?:::::

March 30, 2011 – 2:15 PM

Susan and I sat in an examining room. "This is excruciating," I said to her. "I don't know why I am here. All I know is that I have a couple of bumps on my neck." I reached up and rubbed. "Hopefully we can figure out something today."

"I'm sure we will," she said. "Don't worry so much, it will be fine."

I sat in the examining chair with my head down, rubbing my neck. :::::Maybe if I rub harder.:::::

Knock, knock, knock. The door opened and in stepped Dr. Lee. He was about thirty-five years old, tall and thin, maybe six feet, one hundred and seventy pounds, black hair which didn't touch his ears and brown intelligent eyes. "Hello Stephen, I'm Dr. Lee. How are you doing today?"

"I've been better," I replied. "This is my wife Susan." He looked over and shook hands with her and then looked back at me. "Why am I here?" I said.

"Didn't Dr. Zurbringer call you?" Dr. Lee said.

"He did not. He hasn't called me since he said I might have cancer. He didn't say anything else. He just told me over the phone that I should prepare for the very real possibility that I have cancer and then scheduled me for an ultrasound which I had yesterday."

Dr. Lee seemed somewhat disappointed. "I understand," he said, "I'm sorry Dr. Zurbringer hasn't called you. He is concerned, as am I, that you have these swollen lymph nodes and that they won't go away. Sometimes it means that you may have tongue cancer at the base of the tongue. We can only be sure by performing further tests and observations. Today I want to look down your throat at your tongue using a scope and see what we have."

"Tongue cancer? I don't see anything wrong with my tongue."

"Sometimes the cancer is at the base of the tongue and you can't see it, so you don't have any symptoms. Sometimes the first sign is a swollen lymph node which means that if it is cancer it may have spread to the lymph nodes."

"So you are telling me I may have tongue cancer which may have spread to my lymph nodes? That doesn't sound good."

"It's a possibility, but many times it's something else. Even if I see something on your tongue today, it could be something other than cancer. We'll need to do further tests. Nothing we do today will be definitive."

"Okay"

"Stephen, I'm going to need to take a look. I'm going to spray some stuff in your nose and then we are going to run a tube with a camera through your nose and down your throat. I will need you to relax so I can look at your tongue."

He sprayed a numbing spray into my nose. "I'll be back in a couple of minutes to take a look," he said. He left the room.

"That's not good," I said to Susan. "Tongue cancer which spread to my lymph nodes. That's crazy. I don't feel anything on my tongue. Everything seems normal. I swallow fine, I don't choke on anything. What the hell? How could this be? I quit smoking twenty years ago, I don't chew. I work out. How could I get cancer?"

"He didn't say it was cancer yet. You heard him, it could be a lot of things. Let's find out what is what first." Susan always assumed the best, whereas I always assumed the worst in any given situation.

Dr. Lee came back into the room. "Okay Stephen, let's take a look. Relax." He grabbed a device with a skinny, three feet long, flexible tube on the end of it. The tube was clearly going to go up my nose, over and down to the back of my throat.

"Okay," I said, trying to relax. :::::Sure, you try and relax as somebody is shoving a tube up your nose and down into your throat to find out if you might have cancer. Go ahead, you try to relax.:::::

He shoved the tube up and over into my throat. "Relax," he repeated.

:::::You fucking relax. Please God, let me not have cancer. Please God, please.:::::

He probed around for about five minutes and didn't say anything that I remember. I was praying too hard to hear any voices. After he was done he pulled the tube back out. :::::That hurt.:::::

He looked at me. "Stephen, there is something down there. It's about two by two centimeters. I can't be sure what it is yet."

"Is it cancer?" I asked.

"We can't be sure, but it could be."

"What if it is?"

"Then we can treat it. It's treatable. We have surgery, radiation and chemo which can all be used to treat it."

"Is it curable?"

"It is. But let's do first things first. First we have to make sure we know what it is and if it has spread to your lymph nodes. I'm going to schedule you for a biopsy and a full body scan in the next couple of days.

I can see that you are going to worry, but I want you to know that we are not sure what it is. If it is cancer we can cure it. Do you have any questions?"

"How did this happen? My tongue doesn't feel wrong."

"I don't know Stephen, I really don't. Mrs. Wendt, do you have any questions?"

"No Dr. Lee, I don't."

"When will I have the next test?" I asked.

"I'm going to get you scheduled right away," he said. "Probably on Monday we'll have a biopsy of the lumps on your neck. The doctor will stick you with a needle and take some cells from your lymph nodes to find out what's going on. Any other questions?"

"No," I said.

"You can take a minute and get yourself together and leave when you are ready." He looked me straight in the eye and said, "We'll get through this. I'll see you soon." He promptly left the examining room.

"I can't believe I have cancer," I said, grabbing my neck.

"He said it might not be cancer. He can't be sure and neither can we," Susan said.

"It's cancer, I know it is. You heard him. He's just talking doctor talk. I really like him. I can see he cares about me but he can't say it's cancer, even though he knows that it is. Doctors won't say what something is until they are one hundred percent sure."

"We'll see. One step at a time."

April 4, 2011

Susan and I walked up to the fourth floor of the Sacred Heart Medical Center Clinics in Springfield. I was really getting to hate all these hospitals and medical facilities. It seemed like every day I was getting to visit a new doctor in a new place. It was 8:15 in the morning on Monday. I had dreaded this appointment all weekend and had counted down the hours. I had a hard time sleeping and no matter how much I rubbed my neck the lumps were not going away.

I checked in at the prescribed office and we sat down. Not long after, a man magically appeared in the waiting room. "Steve"

"Yes"

"Right in here please," said the man who held my fate in his hands. He motioned to an open door.

I walked over and crossed through the doorway into some kind of lab. Ahead of me was a metal table. "Have a seat," he said. I did as told. "Okay, today I'm going to look at your neck and stick those lumps with a needle and take out some material. After I get some material out, I'll look at it right here and let you know what's up. Please lie on your side, bumps up."

I lay down, closed my eyes and prayed. First he rubbed my neck with his hands. :::::Dude, I've been doing that over and over. Nothing is going to change unless you have magic hands.::::: About a minute after he started, he stopped and I could hear his chair swivel. I heard him fiddling with something and few seconds later he swiveled the chair back towards me and he used the famous words, "This is going to hurt a little." I braced as he inserted a needle into my neck, moved it around and then pulled it out.

:::::Please Lord, don't let me have cancer, please, please, please.::::: I didn't feel any pain at all, I think I was so nervous that my pain sensors must have shut down. Can you be so worried about something that you feel no pain?

He handed me a cotton ball to put over the now bleeding needle opening. "You can sit up," he said. "I'm going to check the biopsy now."

I sat up and watched as he rolled over to another station. He put some of the material from the needle onto a slide, slid over a few more feet on his metal rolling chair and put the slide under a microscope without saying a word. I watched him adjust the microscope and then put some additional material onto another slide and look it over as well. He sat up and rolled his chair over to me. All in all, it took less than three minutes.

:::::Please don't let me have cancer. I can't have cancer. What did I do to deserve this?:;:::

"I'm sorry Steve, the cells I pulled out are cancerous. Squamous cell carcinoma. It looks like you have cancer of the lymph nodes which probably spread from cancer of your tongue. That happens."

"Are you sure?" :::::Damn it. Damn it. Damn it. What about my family and my kids and my grandkids. I want to see them grow up.:::::

"Yes"

"Is it treatable?" :::::Please say yes, please say yes, please say yes.:::::

"Yes it is. You can beat this. You have cancer in at least two lymph nodes but we can overcome it. Do you have any further questions? I'll give the results to Dr. Lee and you should be seeing him very soon."

"Okay, thanks." Somehow I felt relieved. At least now I knew what I had and now we could make a plan to beat this. I stood up, we shook hands and I walked out the door and looked at Susan. She stood and we walked out of the office together without saying a word. As soon as the office door shut behind me, we stopped and turned toward each other. "He said I have cancer of the lymph nodes but it is treatable."

"I'm so sorry." We looked at each other and hugged. "It is going to be okay, I know it is," she said.

"I hope so." I reached up and rubbed my neck, breaking our hug. We walked slowly towards the car. :::::I can't believe that I have cancer. Why me? What had I done?:::::

April 4, 2011 – 2 PM

Susan and I sat in another one of the examining rooms of the Ear, Nose and Throat Clinic. I looked around. It was so sterile. A couple of pictures that looked like they were stolen from hotel rooms, a couple of $39.95 chairs from a discount office supply store, some drawings of an ear, nose and throat taped up on the wall, just like what you saw in grade school, and a computer sitting on a small stand all surrounded the examination chair and the rolling doctor's stool.

"Now what?" I asked Susan. "I hope they can treat this." It was probably the hundredth time I said those words since learning my fate about five hours ago.

"The other doctor said they could and so did Dr. Lee. Give them some credit."

"I know what they said, but you never know. Some doctors will tell you anything to make you feel better. This could be the end, it's not like a doctor has never said something that didn't turn out to be not true."

"You are jumping to a place you don't need to go."

Dr. Lee entered the room. He did not waste any time. "Okay Stephen, I got the results of your test this morning. As you heard, you have cancer of a couple of lymph nodes in your neck which probably came from the lump on your tongue."

"So I have cancer on my tongue and in my lymph nodes?"

"Probably, but we can't be sure yet. I am going to schedule you for a whole body scan and see what is going on. That way we can tell if it has spread anywhere else. Provided that it hasn't, we need to talk about options."

"What options do I have? Is it treatable?"

"It is, provided it hasn't spread. We can use surgery and also possibly radiation and chemotherapy depending on how serious it is. I am going to get in touch with the cancer institute and we can come up with a plan. First we need to find out the extent of this. Once we do, I am going to do a surgery to get a biopsy of your tongue and then, if it is cancer, I'm going to need to do another surgery to remove the tumor and then another to remove the lymph nodes in your neck. You might also have the option of only radiation and chemo without further surgeries after I biopsy your tongue."

"Three surgeries then possibly radiation and chemotherapy?"

"Yes, but we have to make sure of everything first. I'm going to schedule you for the full body scan first. You should have it this week so we can find out where we are at."

"Okay." Despite my best efforts my voice trembled.

"Steve," Dr. Lee said, "we are going to get through it together and you are going to be okay. Myself, and a lot of other folks, are going to do the best we can to make you better. Hang in there, only a couple more things and we can get a solid plan to get rid of the cancer."

"Thanks Doc, I sure hope so," I said. Susan and I stood up and walked out to our car.

"You are going to be fine." Susan reassured me as we sat in the car. "I like Dr. Lee, he knows what he is doing and really cares. I trust him."

"I do too," I said. "I don't know what to say. Cancer. This sucks." I reached up for my neck praying that the lumps were gone. Still there.

April 7, 2011 – 8 AM

"Okay, Mr. Wendt, here's the drill," a technician said, "I need you to change into a gown in the dressing room and then go to Room 2. When you get there, I'll come in and we'll put some dye into your arm. After that

I'm going to need you to sit back and relax for about twenty minutes. The most important thing is that you don't get upset. Just relax. We'll play some music to help you relax."

"Can you play some AC/DC? I was listening to *Thunderstruck* over and over on the drive over here and it relaxed me."

"Sarcasm?"

"No, for some reason their screaming and the same continuous beat makes me relax. It clears my brain. As my parents would say back in the day, 'It's mind numbing.' I know it's stupid, but that's the way it is. If you want to stress me out, play some elevator music, which will remind me of the music my father listened to and the dentist's office. Those two things will drive my blood pressure up forty points."

"Sorry, no AC/DC. I won't pipe in any music if you hate elevator music, cause that's pretty much all we have. If you get excited it can cause false positives. After about twenty minutes in Room 2, we'll put you in the machine. Once you are in there, I will need you to be very still. We are going to scan from the top of your head to be bottom of your feet. All this should take about an hour and a half and then you can go home. I need you to relax. Got it?"

"Yes, I do." :::::Relax? "Hey dude we are going to look at your whole body and see if your cancer has spread. If it did you might have a death sentence, but chill out and relax!":::::

Thirty minutes later they slid me into the machine. Luckily for me, after serving over twenty years in the United States Navy Submarine Force, it really didn't bother me. It reminded me of the coffin bunks we had on submarines, stacked three deep. You took off your shoes and poopy suit, slid in those little bunks face up and fell asleep. Of all the things that bothered me, small spaces was not one of them.

I didn't fall asleep in this bunk however. I prayed the whole time that I didn't have cancer anywhere else in my body while my eyes darted around following every sound the machine made.

About an hour after they slid me into the machine, they slid me out. A voice from an intercom said, "Okay, Mr. Wendt, that's it. You can get changed and leave whenever you want. Dr. Lee should have your test results within a day."

I silently stood and walked out. I didn't ask the technician what the results were. I had learned my lesson about that. Anything they said would scare me. I was afraid he would tell me to get drunk tonight like I had been told previously. I didn't want any part of that. In actuality, I don't think it would have mattered what he said. If he said everything looked good, I wouldn't believe him and I would be just as afraid as if he said there was somcthing wrong.

April 8, 2011 – 10 AM

Dr. Lee, Susan and I were sitting in the same room where Dr. Lee told me I "might" have cancer. This room made me nauseous, well this room and about ten other rooms, at about four different medical places so far. Everywhere I went, at every medical office, they had rooms which were essentially duplicates of one another, maybe a couple of different pictures. Every doctor's office reminded me of cancer now. I was pretty sure the list wasn't going to get shorter and my feelings weren't going to change anytime soon.

"Okay Steve," Dr. Lee looked at me closely, "good news from the scan. It looks like the cancer is isolated to the two lymph nodes and probably your tongue. It doesn't appear to have spread anywhere else. That's good, so now we know what we are fighting. I can pull up the scan on the computer and you can see what's going on if you want."

The idea of seeing pictures that showed me with cancerous growths in my neck and on my tongue made me seize up. I was not up to seeing cells that were multiplying inside of me at this very moment. :::::How much do you think they have grown since the scan? Double? How about since you discovered the lumps a few months ago? 3X, 4X? They are attacking you. They are trying to spread, maybe they already have. Kill them. Cut them out.:::::

"No thanks doc, I'm not up for that. I believe you. Where do we go from here?" I replied, my voice hiding my fear. Don't let him hear or see your feelings, Steve. Use your training to hold it together. You have experienced life and death emergencies over and over again, this is just another.

:::::No it's not, in those instances you had something to say about the outcome. Not here, you can't control anything here. It's all up to the doctors. Good luck, you're about ready to break down.:::::

"First I need to do a surgery to take a biopsy of the tumor on your tongue. We have the DaVinci machine in Eugene which is good. I sit at a computer and a small device goes down your throat. My hands never go into your mouth, only the machine tip which is controlled remotely by me. I will take a biopsy and see what we have. Once upon a time we had to cut you open from the outside and cause a lot of damage but this machine makes it minimally invasive. If all goes well, you'll be out of the hospital the following day."

"Why can't you just cut the whole thing out, why the biopsy? Just get rid of it."

"I have to make sure it is cancer. We can probably do the biopsy next week."

"We know it's cancer don't we? The MRI says it's cancer, doesn't it?"

"We are ninety-nine percent sure it's cancer, but we can't be totally sure until the biopsy. Hang with me here. We need to follow the established procedures."

"Okay, then what?"

"Then if it's cancer, we have another surgery on your tongue to cut the cancerous portion out, if that's what you want, and then a third surgery to remove the lymph nodes on the left side of your neck. After that, we have to determine if you need radiation and chemo."

"Do I have choices?"

"Two. First, assuming it is cancer, we cut it out and then get radiation and/or chemo if necessary. Second, there is also the possibility that you could possibly go with no further surgery after the biopsy and just have radiation or radiation and chemo."

"What if I want to make sure it's gone? What would you do if you wanted to make sure it was gone?"

"I would get the surgeries and then do radiation and chemo if necessary, but let's see after this biopsy surgery. You don't have to make any decisions yet."

"Okay, set up the surgery." I hung my head.

:::::You didn't fool anyone tough guy.:::::

April 12, 2011 – 7:30 AM

"You'll be fine," Susan said. "It's only a small surgery. No big deal."

"I haven't had any surgery since I was a kid and this is involving my throat. Doctor Lee better know what he is doing and how to operate that DaVinci."

"Dr. Lee knows what he is doing, you're going to be fine."

Susan was driving us to the hospital for the first of my surgeries. I was worried. I was worried about the surgery, I was worried about what they would find. "At least I took care of my will yesterday in case something happens. If something should happen to me you will be taken care of just like we talked yesterday."

"Nothing is going to happen," she said. "You need to keep it together."

"I can't. You know this is the same type of surgery that killed my grandma. She was going in for a biopsy on her neck and the next thing you know we got a phone call telling us she was dead. The doctor nicked her throat and she bled into her lungs. It suffocated her. I can't help but worry."

April 12, 2011 - 2:00 PM

Dr. Lee approached the chair I was sitting in after my surgery. I held my breath.

"Steve, everything went fine."

I exhaled. Thank God he got to the point quick. I was not in the mood for chit-chat.

"We did a biopsy on the area. It is cancer, but it's small enough that we can operate on it without the loss of your tongue. Everything else looked okay down there. The machine worked fine. Next we'll schedule you for second surgery to remove the cancer completely, if that's what you want. Probably next week. You can get out of here tomorrow."

"Schedule it. I want this cancer out of my body."

April 20, 2011 – 10 PM

I wake up and can't swallow. :::::Where am I? My throat hurts. Why is there a tube shoved down my throat? Get it out. Get it out. Hold on, my hands are tied down to the bed. What the hell is going on here?::::: I look over to my right. Susan is there looking at me. I try to say something but all I can do is gurgle.

My wife grabs my hand. "You are okay, everything went okay."

I gurgle again, "Untie my hands. Get this thing out of my mouth." That's what I try to say but it comes out "Unti m and, et ot mou." :::::Damn.:::::

"Nurse, he is trying to say something. I think he wants to be untied and have the tube taken out of his month."

The nurse comes over. I look at her wide-eyed. Dr. Lee said that he might need to put in a tube. He also said that hopefully I could swallow after the surgery. Let me see. I try to swallow, no go. I try again, it works, I can swallow. "I ca wallow." :::::Fuck, I can't get the words out. This damn tube. Take it out!:::::

The nurse turns to my wife. "I'm glad to see he woke up, but I'm going to knock him out again for a while." She grabs a syringe, fills it with some stuff and injects it into the IV. Down I go. :::::NO, NO, NO.:::::

I woke up about five more times that night. One time they loosened my hands (not completely) and gave me a pen and some paper. I tried to write but it came out all scribbly. "I caaaaa szolow" came out for "I can swallow." "I wuv u" came out for "I love you." Susan and the nurse somehow find it funny, I am not amused. Thank God they can't read my mind or understand what I want to say. After a couple of minutes, out comes the needle and they knock me out again. :::::Ha, Ha, Ha.:::::

I wake up about eight the next morning, more clear headed this time. I am still tied to the bed and still have that tube down my throat. They thought if they untied me I would probably go for it. They were absolutely right. I test my swallowing ability again and everything works.

"I'm glad you are awake," my wife said. "You had a rough night. You tried to talk and write but you couldn't."

"Geet dis ot." I point to the tube with my tied down hands. "Geet dis ot." I yank at the restraints. "Unty mo."

She ignores my request. "You are in the ICU, but Dr. Lee said everything went well. He'll be around this morning."

Dr. Lee came around about an hour later. "Get dis out."

"I'll see what I can do." He walks toward the nurses station.

The ICU Doctor is standing outside my room. I hear Dr. Lee ask him to "remove the tube."

The ICU Doctor replies that he can't without permission from the respiratory people and that he doesn't know my status well enough to feel comfortable doing it. :::::Ass, then figure it out quick.::::: Dr. Lee looks over at me and turns to the other doctor.

"I'll take the hit. Pull the tube," Dr. Lee replies.

After a couple of rounds of "I don't know" and "I'll take responsibility," the ICU Doctor finally relents and heads my way.

They let go of the restraints, sit me up and pull the tube. :::::That hurt.::::: I coughed and said, "It's about time. Damn. I can swallow. Can I go home?"

Dr. Lee smiled. "Not yet. Probably tomorrow. We still have the feeding tube in. Everything went well yesterday. I removed a piece of your tongue, we got the necessary clearances and everything should be good. In a couple of weeks we can do the lymph node surgery and in the mean time we'll know what we got. We can get the cancer institute to get a plan together for you for radiation and chemo if necessary. Any questions?"

My head was still clearing up. "No. Thank you. Please get me out of here. I am ready to go home. Thanks for letting me still have a tongue. I can swallow and talk. Get me out of here."

"I'll see you in about a week."

I got moved over to the regular ward an hour later and was up and walking that afternoon. I kept walking until they told me to sit down. First they told me I needed to walk and then they told me to stop walking. Make up your mind. The next day they sent me home.

April 27, 2011 – 10 AM

"Hello Stephen," Dr. Lee said. "How are you feeling?"

"I'm okay," I replied.

"How's the tongue?"

"Pretty much as good as new. It feels a little different and my speech is a little blurry sometimes but good."

"Any trouble swallowing?"

"No, none."

He felt around and ended up at the bumps on my neck. The same place I always ended up.

"Okay, Steve, everything looks good. Next are the lymph nodes. We can do surgery next week. It will require that I cut open the left side of your neck and go in and remove the two lymph nodes. After it heals in a couple of weeks, we can get on with the radiation and chemo if we need it."

"Do I have a choice?"

"You do, we can go straight to radiation and chemo without cutting out the lymph nodes. The radiation and chemo might get rid of the cancer without surgery but the side of your neck will always have those lumps."

"No, cut the damn things out as soon as possible. I don't want to wait any longer. Every time I look at myself in the mirror or touch my neck it reminds me that I have cancer. I need you to get rid of them or they will drive me crazy. I could live with them but I would rather not. What would you do?"

"I would cut them out like you are doing," he said.

"Please let's just get the cancer out of my body. Any residual we can kill out with the radiation and chemotherapy."

"Okay, I'll schedule it for next week. One other thing, I got the bloodwork back from the last tests and you have HPV-16 which is a common factor for this type of cancer. The good news is that it makes it easier to cure."

"What the hell is that?"

"It is a form of herpes. I don't know how you got it but I know that you have it."

I looked at Susan. "Herpes? I haven't had sex with another woman for thirty-six years. So you are telling me that I got a form of herpes thirty-six years ago and it hasn't shown any symptoms or signs for that long until it shows up in tongue cancer? How could that be?"

"I don't know," he said, "but it's there and you have it. I'll schedule you for the surgery next week."

"Thanks, I'll looking forward to it." :::::Really, HPV? How could that be?:::::

A couple of minutes later, I got in the car with Susan. "Really HPV-16?" I said. "I don't understand. How can that be true? It's from something I did when I was sixteen? I got it from a woman in Belize thirty-six years ago and now it shows up as cancer when I am fifty-two? That is ridiculous. How did I even get it?"

"I don't know." Susan looked at me. "You were crazy before you met me."

"Not that crazy. Come on. HPV, thirty-six years ago. What the hell?"

"It also means that you probably gave it to me as well."

"I'm sorry. I have never cheated on you. I swear. I must have got it before we were married."

She didn't say another word. We drove home in silence.

We went home and I looked up HPV-16 on the Internet. There it was. HPV-16 was a common factor in this type of cancer. Once I found it on the Internet, I started looking at everything about the type of cancer I had. Apparently it was Stage Three or Four and the survival rates where about sixty-six percent, higher with HPV. It scared the hell out of me. One out of three people who got this cancer died from it within five years. A bunch also had reoccurrence and sometimes it required removal of all or almost all the tongue. The last thing I looked at were a couple of discussion boards which included people who had the same thing as I had. Some had more than one reoccurrence and others had much of their tongues removed in order to save their lives. That was enough for me. I shut down the Internet and wasn't going back to look at this stuff anymore. I'd seen enough.

Cancer? Stage Three or Four? HPV? HPV-16 causes this? What the hell was going on? Three months ago I was totally healthy, running thirty miles per week and now I'm a wreck. There was a one out of three chance that I wouldn't be alive in five years? A lousy bump that pops up on Valentine's Day turns into this? Why did this happen to me? What did I do to deserve this? Thirty some years ago I get a virus from sleeping with a woman. Thirty some years ago and now it comes out as cancer on my tongue which has spread to my lymph nodes. This is ridiculous. It's so ridiculous that it might just kill me. Plus I probably gave it to Susan. How could I? Maybe I should just ball up and waste away. What good am I? Maybe I'm getting what I deserve.

:::::Enough of that shit.:::

May 4, 2011

"Steve you came out of the surgery fine," Dr. Lee said.

I had just woken up from my third surgery in a month. This one on my neck to remove the cancerous lymph nodes.

"I removed twenty-seven lymph nodes in all. Two had cancer but I removed everything around them as well," he said.

"Twenty-seven?" I replied. "I didn't know you were going for that many."

"I'd rather be safe than sorry. I took out everything around the ones with cancer. I opened up the left side of your neck completely. There are a couple of drains coming out of your neck. We'll take them out in a few days. Here is a mirror." He put it on the bed to my left. "The left side of your neck has about thirty staples in it. We'll remove them in a couple of weeks."

I picked up the mirror and looked at my neck. "Doc, there are staples from my ear to my Adam's Apple. What the hell!"

"It will be okay. They'll come out in a couple of weeks."

:::::Damn, I didn't realize the damage he would be doing. The whole side of my neck had been opened. I looked like Frankenstein. At least I didn't have two big bumps on my neck any longer.::::: "Did you get it all?"

"We did. You can go home in a day or so. Then I'll see you in a couple of days and we'll remove the drains. In two weeks we can remove the staples."

"After that what?"

"I'm going to send everything I have to the Willamette Valley Cancer Institute and they are going to let us know what they can do. You are going to need radiation and probably chemotherapy. I don't know how much. They will evaluate everything and let us know. As soon as they do, I'll let you know."

"Thanks"

"No problem. Feel better. The surgeries are over now. We cut out everything that we could see."

"So I am cancer free now?"

"Possibly, but that's not the way it works. We have to do radiation and probably chemo to make sure that this thing is wiped out. The oncology doctors will let us know what you need. If we stopped now it would probably come back. I highly recommend follow on radiation and chemo."

"Okay. Thanks for doing everything."

"You are more than welcome Steve. I'll see you in a few days."

May 11, 2011

"Okay Steve," Dr. Lee's encouraging voice opened up to me, "everything looks good. I'm going to remove the drainage tubes now. Head up, please."

I bent my head up. He reached over, grabbed a tube and pulled it from my neck. Then, before I had time to react, he did it a second time. "Shit, that hurt."

"I know, it's kind of tender in there, but it looks good. So do the staples. You should be ready to have them out next week."

"Can't you take them out now?" I replied.

"No, sorry. Next week," he continued on. "I talked to the oncology people. Dr. Baker, who is the head of the institute, will be taking your case. It looks like they will need to do thirty-five radiation treatments and three chemo treatments."

"How does that work?"

"You'll have an appointment with Dr. Baker as soon as the staples come out, and he'll let you know the specifics. Basically you'll get one radiation treatment a day for thirty-five days and three chemo treatments over that time. They are going to wear you out, but you are strong and you can handle it."

"Are you sure he needs that much?" Susan said. Her eyes looked startled.

"I think so. If we stopped now it would probably come back without radiation and chemo. The surgeries are over, now we go on to the second half."

"Okay, schedule the appointment as soon as you can." I ended the debate before it started. "I want to get this over with and break its neck."

May 18, 2011 – 2 PM

"Okay, Steve, it looks like everything has healed well. We can remove the staples now. It might hurt a little, sometimes the skin heals onto the staple. Head to the side, so I can remove them please." Dr. Lee reached over for some type of grabbing device. :::::Probably a five thousand dollar staple puller.:::::

I didn't want to see anything else so I closed my eyes and put my head to the side. I was just happy that they were getting the staples out. I felt like a monster. The whole side of my neck was a bunch of staples, all the way down. I had gone out of the house a couple of times in the last week and felt like everyone was staring at me. It was not a comfortable feeling. I heard Dr. Lee snipping away and every once in a while there was a tug and a little pain. The pain was worth it to get rid of these staples.

"Done"

"That wasn't so bad. Thanks."

"You are welcome. Any other issues?"

"Some parts of the side of my neck are numb."

"That's normal. As a matter of fact, you may not get any feeling back in those parts. How have you been doing eating? It looks like you've lost about fifteen pounds since we started."

"I'm taking it easy like you said. Mostly liquids and soft stuff. It feels a little different down there and I'm afraid that the passage is restricted."

"It is a little smaller. Eat what you can. Make sure everything is cut up into small pieces. I spoke to Dr. Baker and you have an appointment later in the week correct?"

"Yes, what can I expect?"

"He's really good and he'll set up what you need to do. This is the last time I'll need to see you until your radiation and chemo are over. After that, I'll see you every other month to make sure everything is okay. You have been doing remarkably well so far. Keep it up."

"Am I going to make it?"

"You are going to make it, Steve. Keep hanging in there." He was smiling at me. "Any other questions?"

"No, but I just wanted to thank you for all you have done." My voice broke up and a tear rolled down my cheek. "You really helped me make it through this. I appreciate it. Thanks for being so great."

:::::So much for holding it together.:::::

"You're welcome. I'll see you soon." He left the room.

:::::Good thing he left before you went full-on boo-hoo.:::::

"Now it's on to the next part. Whoopee," I said to Susan.

"You'll be fine."

"I hope so. I'm not ready to die."

We got up and left the room.

May 20, 2011 - 10 AM

Another day, another doctor's office. This doctor's office was the scariest by far. It was in the Willamette Valley Cancer Institute. Up until we pulled into the parking lot of this place, I still didn't fully comprehend the fact that I had cancer. When we walked up to the building and into the waiting room I so much wanted to turn and run the other way. This could not be happening. Every other doctor's office and medical waiting room is kid's play until you walk into a cancer institute.

The door opened. A man about fifty-five, five feet ten, slim with jet black hair and black rimmed glasses entered the room. "Steve, Susan I am Dr. Baker. I'm here to help you get through this. You have had a lot of work done with Dr. Lee so far and I see you are doing well. We will be helping you get the radiation and chemotherapy you need in order to completely annihilate the cancer. The treatments we are going to give you are very rough. It looks like you will need thirty-five radiation treatments and three chemotherapy sessions. I'm not going to kid you, they are going to wear you down."

"You mean you are going to try and kill any cancer cells without killing me?"

"That pretty much covers it. For the radiation treatments you will be using one of these."

He stood up and reached into a cabinet. He pulled out a mesh mold of a person's torso. "We are going to make a mold of your head and shoulders so we can secure you to a machine and pinpoint the radiation treatments on you. You'll be fitted for the mold next week and we'll probably start treatments by the end of the month. Each treatment takes about fifteen minutes and you'll come in every day, Monday through Friday, to get them. We'll also have follow-up appointments and you'll talk to a nutritionist. The radiation will probably make your throat and mouth so sore that you won't be able to eat regular food. You'll also probably lose your taste, or most of it, possibly forever. Let me take a look at your mouth, throat and neck."

He walked over and looked inside my mouth and felt around my neck for three or four minutes. "Everything looks good. We should be starting by the end of the month. Any questions?"

Dr. Baker was a nice man but he was all business. I had plenty of questions to ask but I was too much in shock to talk about most. "Is this going to kill me?" :::::That cut to the chase.:::::

"It will not." Dr. Baker was subdued. "We will get through this. There will be effects but you can handle them."

"Thanks"

"We'll see you soon Stephen." He exited the room.

I looked at Susan. "This sounds like fun. But I guess it's what we need to do to survive. I hope I live through it. I saw on-line that sometimes people die from this."

"You'll be fine." She stared out the window at the trees outside.

I prayed she was right. "We have to see to the Chemo Doctor now."

May 20 ,2011 - 11 AM

The Chemotherapy Doctor's appointment was a blur. He seemed to be preoccupied with my fingernails. I have no idea why. He looked like he was about twelve years old but at that point I didn't care. I was in for the ride, tell me what I need it do and I will do it. He let me know that I would be receiving three treatments. One at the beginning of radiation, one in the middle and one at the end. He said it was some type of platinum treatment which would kill the bad cells. He also said each treatment would be about four to five hours and they would make me tired and probably nauseous. He also let me know that I might be losing my hair, but probably not. The side effects where everything from feeling like I had a common cold to death.

:::::Nice. That about covers it.:::::

I just wanted to get out of there. I didn't have much choice but to do it and try to make it through. I'd been dealing with this shit for almost three months already and I had almost two weeks before my radiation and chemo started. I just wanted to forget for a little while before they started on me again. I just wanted to forget. :::::Good luck with that.:::::

I opened my eyes.

:::::Here I am in the Chemo Treatment Room. Yuch.:::::

I looked at Susan and we smiled at each other.

"Only a couple of hours left. You have been out for about two hours," she said.

I drank lots of water for the next couple of hours and used the bathroom a few times, rolling my bag of magic poison behind me. Other than that I did not talk much. I tried to watch television (there was one attached to the chair) and read but I couldn't concentrate. Susan tried to talk with me but I wasn't interested. She went out and got me some juice and something to eat but I wasn't hungry. My eyes continually locked on that damn bag, dripping the brown liquid. I kept waiting for something bad to happen.

By four o'clock in the afternoon I was home. Exhausted. Probably from the fear more than from the radiation and chemo. I was waiting for my body to revolt against me since my mind was already in a full-on revolt.

Day 2 – Wednesday - June 1, 2011

We pulled into the lot of the cancer institute which was situated on Country Club Road, directly across from the Eugene Golf Club. It sat back from the road, tranquilly hidden in plain sight. Only a small sign on the road with the predominant letters WVCI and the ultra-small letters Willamette Valley Cancer Institute gave it away. I had probably driven by the sign thirty times before all this started and I had no idea that it was for a cancer institute. Maybe I didn't pay attention or maybe I didn't want to know, but I knew where it was now.

We couldn't park in the front row of the parking lot. All the spaces were handicapped spots. I suppose I could get a placard, but plenty of patients were much worse off than me. They could use them. :::::I'm not that sick. Parking there means I semi-give up.:::::

Susan parked in a spot a couple of rows back. "How about we skip it today," I said. I really didn't have any intention of not going but I was letting her, and myself, know how much I hated being here. :::::Like we needed any reminder.:::::

"It's 8:15 and I have to go see the nutritionist before I go in for my radiation treatment. What are they going to tell me? Eat more?"

"You've lost about seventeen pounds since this started," Susan voiced her concern. "Plus you didn't eat much this morning or yesterday after we got home."

"I'm okay. The chemo upset my stomach. I drank some milk and had some oatmeal this morning. I was able to keep it down. I'll be fine. I mean really, look at me, I could lose fifty pounds before I get skinny. I weigh about two hundred and thirty pounds right now."

"Yeah, but you started at two hundred and forty something, almost two hundred and fifty, only a couple of months ago. You have to eat."

"Tell it to the chemo and radiation, I don't think they are going to do a lot for my appetite."

We got out of the car and headed in. I paid my twenty-four dollars at the counter. Twelve for the radiation and twelve for the nutritionist. Five minutes after we arrived we were in the nutritionist's office.

"Stephen, I'm Celeste, your nutritionist. During this process we are going to monitor your progress and make sure you are doing okay. Typically as the treatment goes on you will get less hungry. Your mouth and throat are going to get sore and dry and you may not want to eat but I need you to get calories in. I don't want you losing more than fifteen or twenty pounds during the next seven weeks and that means you have to get calories in. You are going to weigh in every week and we'll see how it goes."

"Eating is easier said than done. I got some oatmeal down this morning, but frankly the radiation and chemo I received yesterday has me down a little bit. I have some nausea, I'm tired and I really don't care if I am eating right now."

"That's normal, but you are only one day into it. I need you to eat as much as you can during the next few weeks because after that it's going to get more difficult to get things down. At some point you may have to switch over to protein drinks or we can always put in a feeding tube."

"No tube, no way. I'll get the food down. I'm not getting a tube to feed me. I've had it with operations and I don't want any more unless I absolutely need them. No tube." :::::No way.:::::

"Got it. No tube. Then do yourself a favor and eat. Eat healthy but bring in the calories. Some of the protein drinks are pretty good. You'll be able to taste them now, but in the near future your taste buds are going to get wiped out from the radiation. That will probably happen in the next week or so."

"I already lost some of my taste after the tongue surgery."

"I know, but it will most likely get worse. Keep your head up and get through this."

"Okay." I gave a half-smile which I don't think she believed for a second. "I'll get through it."

I looked at her for the first time. Until that time, she was just another face in the crowd of treatment faces. She was about fifty and thin. Reminded me of Mrs. Osterhaus, my fifth grade teacher, the crankiest teacher I ever had. :::::What did you expect from a nutritionist?::::: Wore glasses, had brown hair, almost down to her collar. "I'll be honest with you," I said, "I am kind of using this to lose a few pounds. Look at you. You are healthy right? You are thin. I could lose a few pounds."

"Bad idea. Now is not the time to go on a diet. We can't have you losing too much weight too fast. You need to keep your energy. Yesterday was just the start. You need your energy to fight."

:::::Whatever.::::: "Okay, I'll do my best."

"Oh, and no supplements or gimmicky stuff. No miracle cures or Eastern remedies. None. I know there is a lot of stuff available that's supposed to make you feel better during chemo and counter the effects of the chemo and radiation but don't get it and don't take it. Take the prescriptions we give you and that's all. I don't know if some of those things work, but I do know they can mess up the necessary effects of the chemo and radiation. We need both to do their work fully. If you want to take some kind of supplement or something like that, you need to talk to me and your doctor first. Generally the answer will be NO. Get it?"

"Got it."

"Any other questions?"

"No"

"Mrs. Wendt, do you have any questions?"

"What should I do if he doesn't want to eat? Any suggestions?"

"You can visit me and we'll see if both of us together can change his mind."

"Sounds like a plan."

I turned to Susan. "What are you going to do, tell on me?"

"Yes I am. It's your health we are talking about. Like Celeste said, you need your energy."

"So you are on a first name basis now?"

"Yes," both said in unison.

Celeste turned back to me, and reached for her desk with her right hand, pulling a couple of business cards. She handed one to both my wife and myself. "Either one of you can come and see me anytime. Steve, if you're having problems eating or something doesn't feel right, let me know."

"Thanks," I said.

Celeste stood and walked out of the room. "That was fun," I said to Susan. "What is that? You are going to tattle on me if I don't eat? I am not getting a tube. No, I am not. I will do whatever it takes to not get a tube."

"You heard her. You better eat as much as you can now."

It was 8:55 when we left the nutritionist and headed out into the corridor. At the intersection of WAITING ROOM and TREATMENT ROOM, I took a right towards my locker and Susan took a left to the waiting room.

By 9 AM I was in my designated place at my designated time. The treatment waiting cubicle had six chairs and a couple of end tables with mostly chick magazines. *Redbook*, *Cosmopolitan*, *Woman's Day*, and a *Reader's*

Digest. No sports magazines here. I looked over at the stack and tried to figure out what I was looking at yesterday but I had no idea. :::::I hope it wasn't *Cosmo* or *Woman's Day*.::::: I'm going to have to put in a complaint that there isn't enough stuff for men. Maybe they could get a subscription to *Sports Illustrated* or *ESPN the Magazine,* perhaps *Golfer's Digest.* Well at least they had a *Reader's Digest.* I was here with the same four ladies as yesterday. One was reading a real book made of paper, another was reading a Kindle, a third was knitting and the fourth stared straight ahead, appearing to be pissed off. I could understand the pissed off one, I don't know how the other three could concentrate waiting for their appointments.

"How many do you have left?" the knitter said.

"Who me?" I said.

"Yes." She smiled. "How many treatments do you have left? You came in yesterday for the first time, I think, but it was clear that you didn't want to say much. All four of us have been doing this for a few days. Pam has eighteen left, Joan has thirteen left, Michelle has twenty-two left and I have only nine more treatments to go. How many do you have left?"

"Thirty-four."

Even the pissed off one looked toward me after I said that. The knitter said, "Ouch, that's a lot. What for?"

"Tongue and lymph node cancer."

"Joan and I are here for breast cancer, Pam has ovarian cancer and Michelle is here for something in her stomach. We've been meeting here every day for a while. Where are you from?"

"Right down the road in Springfield, about ten miles away."

"That's not bad. We come in from the coast every morning. Leave there at 6:30 and get here at 8:30 or so for our treatments, then we go back home."

"You have to ride a bus four hours a day?"

"Yep, but it's better than not riding. What choice do we have? They said that this will make us better, so here we are, getting better."

A technician came in and called Pam's name. She stood up and followed him as ordered.

"By the way, I'm Eileen," the knitter said as she stuck her skinny hand out. We shook. "Good luck," she said and smiled.

"Same to you," I said with the tinge of a smile. The first real one I had for a while.

I was next. "Steve," my technician said. I stood and followed.

I stared down the machine, looking at the opening which the upper part of my body, bound by mesh and bolts would soon be jammed into. I considered walking away.

:::::Man up.:::::

Eileen didn't look like she was here feeling sorry for herself and she was getting multiple treatments for breast cancer, plus she had to ride a bus four hours a day to get this done. Here I was feeling sorry for myself. She must have been five foot nothing and weighed less than one hundred pounds and she could still smile. It was easy to see that she was having a hard go of it. She had a bandana on, the international cancer call sign for loss of hair, and seemed very tired, but the life was in her eyes. She was fighting. :::::Screw you machine.:::::

I sucked it up, finished my trek, assumed the horizontal position and waited. I must have hit my marks perfectly as the technician, dressed in scrubs with some ridiculous pattern, didn't say a word when he bolted me in. When he finished strapping me in he said, "Okay you are ready for take-off. I'll be back in fifteen minutes. Do you need any music?"

"No, thanks," I said, closing my eyes tightly. I did not want to look at this machine that was trying to kill me.

At the first hum of the machine I began to count to get my mind off what the machine was doing to me. One Mississippi, two Mississippi. My thoughts soon went to my daughter Stephanie, who called me last night from Hawai'i.

"Mom, Dad, I don't feel good, I don't want to go bowling."

We were in the parking lot of the bowling lanes in Kempsville, Virginia. "Come on Stephanie, it's a day off and we need to do something," I said. "You haven't been feeling all that well lately and maybe bowling will help. You're twelve years old and you need to get out and do something. Did you eat the sandwich Mom made for you?"

"I told you I don't feel good, I'm thirsty. Mom, please don't make me go bowling. I just want to go home."

I pushed. "Come on Stephanie, we are going bowling, like it or not. Get out of the car and let's go. It's my first day off the ship for a while. Let's have some fun."

"I don't feel good."

"Get out, let's go." I was exasperated.

"Dad we don't have to go. Stephanie doesn't feel good," Steve, our eight year old son, said.

"Let's go home," Susan said. "Maybe I should take her to the doctor. She hasn't been feeling well for a while."

"I don't think it's right. Everyone is ready to have a good time. We haven't done anything together as a family for a while and it would be good to do something together."

"Dad, I'm sorry, I really don't feel good," Stephanie said.

I put the car in reverse, backed out of the spot and headed back home.

"You take care of Steve," Susan said a couple of minutes after we got back home. "I'm taking Stephanie to the emergency room right away. Something is wrong. She's always thirsty and never hungry. She hasn't felt good for a week or so. It's not like her."

Less than an hour later I got a call from Susan. She and Stephanie were getting in an ambulance and were on their way to St. Luke's Hospital in Norfolk. "It looks like Stephanie has diabetes," she said.

"Diabetes?"

"Yes, diabetes. Her blood sugar is screaming high right now and she is breathing erratically. They have an IV in her. It looks like she will be okay. We are lucky we took her to the emergency room when we did. Any longer and she could have died."

I was in shock. How could my little girl have diabetes? What the hell caused that?

They got Stephanie's blood sugar under control and the next week was spent teaching her and Susan and I to manage her Type 1 Juvenile Diabetes, the kind that never goes away no matter what you do. The best prognosis we got was that maybe in ten or fifteen years they would find a cure.

:::::No such luck. It's been twenty-two years now and still no cure. She lives with it every day.:::::

At twelve she followed all the rules, taking her blood sugar three or four times a day and giving herself shots, but by the time she was fourteen she was beginning to rebel by not taking her blood sugar as often as she should and not giving herself the shots she needed. She would eat the foods she shouldn't and her blood sugar would go screaming high into the three and four hundreds when it should have been from eighty to one hundred and twenty.

High blood sugars were bad but the scariest times were when she would have low blood sugar. On one occasion Stephanie, who was fifteen or sixteen at the time, had been watching her brother and sister, while Susan and I went to a movie. When we came home I went into the TV room and saw her lying there, barely breathing, her eyes wide open and dilated. I thought she might be dead. I have never been more afraid in my life, not even when the doctor told me I had cancer. We gave her an emergency shot and ten minutes later she pulled out of it, but she put the fear of God into me with that episode. Day after day, after that, for years on end, I woke up in the middle of the night and went into her bedroom to make sure she was okay. I would shake her, ask her a question and not leave until I received a coherent answer.

On more than one occasion her answers were not coherent and I would try to get some food and sugar into her. She would lay on the floor and thrash and scratch, totally out of it, not wanting to eat or drink. Once we got some sugar into her she would become the sweetest person you could ever know, but when she had low blood sugar she was a terror. It wasn't her fault, it was the damn disease's fault.

When she was nineteen or twenty, I got a call from her about two in the morning and it was clear she didn't know where she was and then she hung up on me. For the next thirty minutes she wouldn't answer my calls. Eventually she called and explained the situation. Apparently when she was driving her blood sugar went low and she instinctively went to a drive-thru window at McDonalds for a soda. When she got it, she sipped some and called me, but her blood sugar wasn't high enough yet for her to be totally coherent, so she hung up and I panicked, not knowing what to do until she called back.

It's a miracle that she didn't have an accident.

I fear for her life every day. When the phone rings in the middle of the night the first thing I think is: "God please let everyone be okay. Please let Stephanie be okay." I am scared senseless that my little girl, who is in her thirties now, won't be okay.

At twenty-one she had a little boy, my grandson Stuart, and at twenty-seven she had a two pound baby boy at thirty weeks. :::::That's right, two pounds at thirty weeks.::::: If her pregnancy had gone on any longer Stephanie would not have survived, the diabetes was causing such havoc on her body. Stephanie and that little guy, Charles, both made it through, thank God. The doctor told her, "No more children."

Stephanie is now the happiest person I know. She faces her diabetes every day and fights. Behind all that happiness lives one tough person. She is tougher than anybody I ever served with in my twenty-eight years in the Navy. There is no way that her illness can be easy for her. There is no let up from it. Ever. The diabetes doesn't take a day off, it doesn't go away. There are no cures for it. :::::Maybe someday.:::::

For the past twenty years, I have never heard her complain about her disease. She doesn't blame anybody. She lives a full and normal life except that she sticks herself with needles multiple times a day and has to make sure that her blood sugar is always good, day and night. She has given herself thousands and thousands of insulin shots all over her body and has taken her blood sugar tens of thousands of times.

If she can do this so can I. :::::SUCK IT UP, BUTTERCUP.:::::

I opened my eyes and watched as the machine circled, rattled and hummed - trying to kill the bad before it killed me. I closed my eyes again and concentrated on getting rid of the noise. :::::No such luck.:::::

Eventually the machine stopped. I opened my eyes and looked up at the device and it looked down at me, asleep. I was done for the day.

Day 3 – Thursday - June 2, 2011

I took a pill for nausea last night and another one this morning. After chemo, they told me that on day two or three it would be the worst. I figured they were just talking doctor talk, but not so this time. Somehow I had denied that the chemo would get to me. :::::Oops, I was wrong.::::: It wasn't so bad, it was like having a mild case of the flu. Feeling sweaty was followed by feeling frozen then back to sweaty. Tired and more tired. Nauseous. I had to sleep with my head raised up to feel semi-okay and not throw-up. It wasn't bad if you didn't eat.

At least I wasn't losing my hair. I combed my hair about five times a day to see if any strays were coming out. A few were, but I don't think those were more than normal.

"Jeez, I hate the weather here," I said to Susan on the way to the clinic. "It's always wet and rainy and in the sixties. Where is summer? It should have been here last month. It's day after day of rain. How long has it been raining, seven months? Enough already. It's June, come on."

"It's been better. It's warming up. We're supposed to have better weather in a couple of days. Maybe the weekend."

"I am so tired of this. I need some sun and some heat. Our house built in the middle of the woods doesn't help. Even when there is sun, there is no sun on us. We are surrounded by those damn trees and the sun can't make it through. What was it advertised as? Filtered light? Whatever. Tell me again why we left Hawai'i and moved here?"

"This place is probably saving your life. It's the best for us. There is no clinic like this in Hawai'i with all the advanced equipment. Be glad we are here."

"I know, but it doesn't feel like the best for me. We come here and a few months later I am dealing with this shit."

"You're just upset today."

"You are damn right I am. We are in a place without many friends, most of our family is in Hawai'i, and the weather sucks. What is there to like?"

Susan drove silently the rest of the way. I shouldn't have said a damn thing. It was just the weather, it couldn't be controlled. It wasn't her fault. :::::Cut it out, dipshit. And it's only day three.:::::

We parked in the lot, got out of the car and silently walked towards the clinic. Ahead of us was an older man in a wheelchair with a woman pushing him along. There were also a couple of people standing out in front of the building smoking. :::::Smoking? Smoking? Are you kidding me? This is a Cancer Clinic and they are smoking outside?::::: One of the smokers was an associate from the waiting room. :::::It takes a real woman to look cancer in the eyes and light up a cigarette.::::: I veered away from the smokers as we moved to within a couple of feet of the door which automatically slid open to suck us in.

Once inside, I followed my daily routine of checking in and paying my twelve dollars, dropping of Susan in the waiting area and heading into the changing room. I was not in the mood for any of it today.

"Okay Steve, buckle up," the technician, dressed in tie-dye scrubs, said to me. "This will be day three right? Only thirty-two to go after this one."

I didn't say a word and got into the dreaded position. :::::Yeah, only thirty-two more days of this!!!:::::

He left me alone and bolted me in. "See you in a few. I left on the radio."

Nothing to be said in reply, I just closed my eyes. Some song on the radio ended and Santana came on singing *Oya como va* which means: "Hey, how's it going?"

:::::How's it going? How's it going? I'll tell you how it's going. Like crap. That's how it's going. I feel like shit and I gave my wife a hard time. I am such an idiot.:::::

I had just opened the bar at my father's hotel, El Pescador, situated on the island of Ambergris Caye, about three miles from the town of San Pedro in Belize. It was Christmas Eve, the 24th of December 1975. After three years of planning and building, the hotel was finally finished and this was the first Christmas with guests. I hated it at the hotel. I hated it because my parents and I did not get along. I was seventeen and I wanted to do whatever I wanted without consequence. I was here, away from exile, for a couple of weeks.

THE LOOKING MASK

When I was in exile I attended Wesley College, really a high school, in Belize City, about thirty-six miles from our hotel by boat. Those miles by boat made it far enough away that I only visited the hotel every few months while going to school.

I'd been exiled because my father and mother couldn't handle me any longer. I was a young man out of place or maybe I was a child in the wrong place. Three years earlier, my father had picked up everything and moved us from Sussex, Wisconsin to this island. I was fourteen years old and had just begun high school when he moved us. He made me leave my friends, my sports, and the place I had grown up in to come here.

When we got here we had no electricity, no running water, no TV, one radio station and a twenty-by-twenty foot house, if you could call it that, which wasn't finished. It had no bathroom or kitchen. We essentially camped out for about three months.

I had no friends and I didn't speak or understand the local language, Creole.

All that changed rapidly. I learned to love San Pedro. Within a few months I was speaking Creole and I had a girlfriend who was Mayan and Creole. My parents, who moved us here to get away from the United States and the rat race, strongly disliked who I had become and tried to make me speak English "correctly" as well as not have a girlfriend. :::::What did they expect, I was a kid.::::: By the time I was sixteen I had dropped out of school, turned into a runaway and become a lobster fisherman.

About a year after I ran away from home my parents and I had come to a truce. They knew I couldn't live with them at the hotel permanently, nor did they want me to, since El Pescador was close enough to town that I could walk to see my girlfriend when I wanted. I knew I couldn't live with them for longer than a couple of weeks at a time without getting into a fight with my father and mother over my girlfriend, so I was sent to Belize City to go to school. While at school I lived in the Bellevue Hotel and tended bar even though I was only seventeen.

It worked out for them. I wasn't the family embarrassment I had become to them in San Pedro.

Soon after my arrival at the hotel for Christmas break, Mrs. Wainright, our next door neighbor, who lived about a half-mile down the beach warned me that her daughter, Susan, would be visiting for Christmas and that I "would love her." I didn't believe it. My girlfriend in town took all my time and energy when I was here and had done so for over two and one half years.

The guests of the hotel and my family had just finished consuming the fishing village Christmas Eve Dinner of lobster and shrimp and everyone was in the mood to have a good time, except for me. I just wanted to do my mandatory service of bartending for a couple of hours and then go to town to attend the dance and be with my girlfriend. My father promised that we would shut down the bar early and take a boat to town around eight or nine.

At 7:26 on that Christmas Eve all that changed. It changed from the very moment that she walked through the hotel's mahogany doors and entered the bar. Everything, as far as a girlfriend was concerned, had seemed so simple and so right until that very minute. At the very moment she entered my brain went haywire.

She was a sight. She stood about five foot-eight and weighed about one hundred and thirty pounds. She wore a white sleeveless blouse and pink short shorts. She had blue eyes and dishwater brown hair. She smiled at me with gleaming teeth as she headed towards the bar and sat down, "*Tequila Sunrise*, please," she said. "Without the tequila." She winked at me, and looked at her mother who trailed immediately behind her with her father.

I knew what that meant. We were both seventeen and there was no drinking age in Belize. Either her parents, Mr. and Mrs. Wainright, weren't looking or they were looking the other way or they didn't care because they were in a hurry to have something to drink as well. It didn't matter to me. What did matter to me was that she knew what a *Tequila Sunrise* was and that she winked and smiled at me. I would have given her anything she wanted. I quickly got her mother and father a round of drinks and sent them on their way. I poured Susan the *Tequila Sunrise* with Tequila and handed it over.

"*Tequila Sunrise* at sunset," I said.

She laughed at the first words I spoke to her and said, "Thank you." She raised the glass to her red face, it had been burned by the first day of Belizean sun which the winter in New York had not prepared her for, and took a sip. "Whoa, that's some strong orange juice. Just the way I like it."

"No problem, I puts in extra Grenadine. I'm Steve."

"I know. I heard all about you from my mother. I'm Sue."

"I heard all abouts you from your mother as well. She say I would love you."

She laughed again and flashed me those perfect white teeth. How could I not be overcome by this girl? My brain and body were in an uproar. :::::You have one girlfriend. You no can do this.::::: Despite the fact that my brain was telling me not to spend time with her, I was doing it anyway. Brain be damned, body be damned. This was chemistry.

"My mother also said that you would be trouble," she said.

"You no can believe everyting you hears."

She laughed at me again. "You sound like you are from here."

"You mom forget to tell you dat I speak dis way? I speak dis way cause dis is where I from. Why you speak da way you speak? Why you speak like you from New York?"

"I am from New York."

"Well der you goes," I said.

She laughed. "Don't worry, I like your accent."

"And I likes yours," I said. "You know I have one girlfriend right?"

"So my mom said. I have a boyfriend as well. In New York." She drained her drink and put the glass down on the bar.

"I guess we be even den." I reached over, grabbed her glass and made her another drink with extra tequila, making sure nobody was watching.

"I guess so. What's going on here?" She looked around the dining area and bar of the hotel at the thirty or so people who were in conversation and listening to Sergio Mendes, much to my chagrin. I loathed Sergio Mendes, probably just because my father liked him. Clearly the guests were getting in a good mood.

"All da gringo's getting drunk. Dat's what is going on. All I knows is dat in an hour or so, by nine, I gots to get going to town, to da dance and to my girlfriend."

"My mom says we're going to town for the Midnight Mass."

We continued to talk. She was so beautiful and engaging that I thought twice about going to town but I had to go. My father walked up to Susan and me about eight forty-five.

"Steve, it looks like you are having a great time. How about you just stay here with us and we not go to town. The party is right here."

"No, I gots to go. You said we go at nine. It's almost nine now."

"I don't think we are going to go," he said, and then turned and moved back into the crowd.

I turned to Susan. "I gots to deal with dis crap all da time. He promised we go to town and now we no going. I going for walk."

"Walk? Are you kidding me? It's pitch dark outside and almost three miles to town. What about the river? You have to swim it."

"Dat's okay, I do it all da time. It no big deal."

"You don't have to go yet do you?" she said.

I was so tempted to stay. :::::Look at her. Look at her. She is da most beautiful girl you ever see and you are saying no to staying with her. You know what for happened when she walked in da door. You almost collapsed you dummy. Stay.::::: "I no can stay, sorry. Maybe I see you in town for da Midnight Mass. I gots for go."

"Will I see you again? I'll be here for a couple of weeks," she said.

"We see," I said, topping off her drink once more. That would be four drinks in about an hour and one half. Ouch.

She flashed those teeth and those blue eyes looked at me again. :::::Mon, dis could screw everyting up.:::::

"I hope so," she said.

I ran to town in the pitch dark, along the edge of the slowly lapping water. Ironically my mother and father, as well as Susan, her parents and a bunch of hotel guests, sped by me in a couple of boats just as I made it to the edge of town about 9:15. I saw Susan at Midnight Mass as I sat with my girlfriend a couple of rows back. Susan and I shared glances with each other a few times during mass. She later told me that the nativity scene seemed all blurry during the mass. She was pretty drunk by the time she got there. :::::I wonder why.:::::

Sitting next to my girlfriend during that mass all I could think about was Susan, her eyes, her smile and her laugh.

Two nights later Susan and I kissed on the dock of El Pescador.

The humming stopped and I opened my eyes. The red lights blinked and laughed at me, and a second or two later the technician entered the room and unbolted my restraint.

I got out of there without saying a word, quickly changed and headed for the waiting room.

There she was. We were both fifty-two now, but when I looked at her today she was still eighteen. :::::Why had I been such an ass for the last years?::::: When I looked at her I knew that I still loved her. :::::Why did I sometimes act like a jerk? I love her, why didn't I show it like I should? ::::: She stood up and we walked out to the car together.

"How did it go?" she asked.

"I love you."

"I love you too." She started the car and Sirius Channel 32 – the Bridge – music from the seventies came on. Elton John started singing *Goodbye Yellow Brick Road.* Any conversation we were about to have ended and we both listened.

:::::You're not in Oz anymore Steve.:::::

I never answered Susan's question.

Day 4 – Friday - June 3, 2011

Yesterday evening I made a vow to myself and today I'm keeping it by full-on watching the machine rotate around me for the first time. Red lights, green lights, red light, more red lights, slowly spinning. It's like a comic book death-ray machine from outer space shooting invisible rays into my head and neck. My eyes, a couple of the only things I can move from my shoulders on up, are following the sometimes steady, mostly blinking lights. This mesh cast is so tight on me I can't even wiggle my ears. I can, however, flare my nostrils and move my lips to scream if I want to. Hopefully I'll never have to do the later, although I've come close to it a couple of times already.

I defiantly flare my nostrils over and over to show the machine who's in charge. Despite its best efforts, it cannot stop me from doing what I want. :::::Yeah right, fire too much radiation into me and it will stop me from doing everything that I want forever.:::::

Today, for the first time, other than our cursory introductions, I talked to my crazy scrub technician. I learned that his name is Mike. Mike Smith. :::::I wonder if that's his name or if he just says it is?::::: He's about the same height as me, about ten years younger, and probably twenty pounds less than me. Maybe two hundred and ten pounds. :::::By the end of this you will probably catch up to him.::::: He has curly red hair and blue eyes. Always ready to smile. Seems to always wear anything but the standard blue or green medical scrubs. Today he has on a Grateful Dead Dancing Bear pullover scrub top. :::::He's from Eugene, what do you expect.:::::

If I had his job I would probably call myself Mike Smith as well. Five days a week dealing with sick people eight or however many hours a day. All day, fifteen minutes each person, thirty-two per day, one hundred and sixty per week. What's that, about eight thousand treatments per year? I don't know how he does it. :::::I'd want to forget my own name if I walked in here every day, day after day.::::: I'd want to forget my name and who I was until my shift was over and I could throw Mike Smith into my locker, hopefully one with permanent signage, along with my dancing bear medical scrubs until the next day. It must take a special kind of person to do this every day. You have got to have your mind right in order to look into the eyes of people who have a good chance of being dead soon.

Every time I walk into this institute it feels so sterile and reeks of despair and lavender, which I have suddenly grown an aversion towards, lavender that is. I don't know where I got the aversion from, but whenever I smell lavender it triggers something unconscious inside of me. I have to leave the area when I smell it. It never used to bother me, but this morning I asked Susan to remove everything which smelled of lavender from the house. It sucks because it's one of her favorite smells. :::::I should have known.:::::

I stopped to look at the institute gift store today on my way to the locker room. They have t-shirts for sale at the gift store that say HOPE in big capital letters. It is so hard to fulfill the promise of the t-shirts when you see everyone around you. :::::Can you believe they have a gift store in a cancer institute? T-shirts, Teddy Bears, flowers. Are you kidding me? "Honey, look what I bought the kids, I got it at the cancer institute today." Not me, I want nothing to remind me of this place.:::::

The non-treatment waiting areas of this place are so medicinally sterile, the same chair after the same chair after the same chair, all with the same greenish-yellow flowery sickly pattern. Where there isn't a chair there is a double chair, same pattern, where there isn't a chair or a double chair there are flimsy tables, all exact duplicates made of cheap laminate. In the middle of both the main waiting rooms, radiation and chemo, there are four-seat game tables, each equipped with the mandatory thousand piece, nearly impossible, jigsaw puzzle with a tree or flower motif, :::::Probably lavender.::::: two or three corners complete and a bunch of individual pieces in the middle of the table scattered about. :::::Every time I see those puzzles I have the sneaking desire to steal an edge piece or two. Just kidding. That would be mean and I'm not into mean right now.:::::

No TVs in the waiting rooms here, no ESPN or CNN or FOX to burn time, only those puzzles and *Reader's Digest, Woman's Day, Redbook* and *National Geographic* magazines to look at while you wait for your at-bat or wait for the person you are with who is currently having his/her swings at the plate.

I'll give them this, they move people in and out on schedule. There is no waiting for hours in the waiting rooms here. Everything is done on time, with precision.

Outside the waiting room, behind every door, except for the gift shop, was my own personal dread. Behind every door was the potential of devastation. Behind most of the doors were doctors or machines. The machine's scared the hell out of me but the doctors scared me a lot more. Every time the doctors spoke I was waiting for them to tell me that there was nothing more they could do for me.

Both the doctors and the machines are trying to fix me by killing part of me. I am having a hard time grasping the concept. :::::For all you know today they are shooting at nothing, just wrecking cells that should not be wrecked.:::::

Thank God it's Friday.

I'm only four days into it and I feel okay, but as Doctor Baker repeated to me today, at my fifteen minute 8:30 AM appointment, "It has a cumulative effect over you. This week you had chemotherapy and radiation for four days and your body is reacting to those treatments. You should be feeling tired, soon your throat will be getting sore and it will be harder to eat, you'll lose most of your taste and get more and more fatigued. You need to keep eating and resting. You are doing fine."

:::::I'm doing fine. Did I have a choice? I'm not going to give up. Put me in coach, I'm ready to play centerfield. No, make that I'll be the catcher. You pitch whatever you have to pitch and I'll be caged in, catching whatever you send my way. I've been practicing my whole life.:::::

Mike Smith, the technician, looked a lot like Bob Jones. :::::Man, does that sound stupid. Bob Jones – Mike Smith.:::::

Bob Jones was gone now, I heard he had died from brain cancer but he once changed my life at the El Pescador Bar in September 1976.

"Steve do you want to play a game of dice? I'm bored here. How about we play a game of Ship's, Captain and Crew?" Bob was sitting on the end of the bar in the same seat Susan sat on when she came in the door almost a year previously. It was about eight o'clock at night, maybe it was 7:26, my own personal magic time. Two couples were sitting at the bar along with Bob. They were wrapped up in themselves, conversation and *Rum and Cokes* with a slice of lemon. I pretty much left them alone, checked on them every fifteen minutes or so to make sure they had plenty to drink and let them do their thing.

"No Mon, I no gots no money," I said.

"We'll play for a couple of bucks. You can afford that can't you? I have to do something here, it's a long way from Nevada."

Bob had moved to Belize from Nevada a few months previously. His story was stranger than most stories of people who moved to an island in Belize, and that was saying something. Within four miles of us was a guy who helped develop RADAR, another who invented the flip-top tab, another who went bust in the oil business, someone who was an animal trainer who trained the MGM lion and a few people who "had it" with the American way of life and had "bagged it." You could put my father in that last category.

Bob's story was that he had opened a house of ill repute in Nevada. He started it with a couple of trailers and it doubled in size every year. :::::Imagine that, there was apparently a call for ladies of the night in Nevada, the home of sin.::::: He built his business into one of the largest cat houses in Nevada and about a year ago a couple of gentlemen walked up to him in his establishment and made him an offer for his property and business even though it wasn't for sale.

It was a substantial offer with a fair price, but Bob said, "No Thank You," knowing that his business would continue to grow. A couple of days later the two original gentlemen, along with a new gentleman, brought him a larger check and told him it was a "final" offer. Bob asked, "What if I say no?" He was promptly told that he did not want to say "No" because this was a "final offer" in more ways than one.

Bob politely took the offer from the "gentlemen," cashed the check and asked no further questions. He disappeared to Ambergris Caye with his wife and a much younger woman. Neither was there with him that night. :::::Even former owners of brothels needed a break or got kicked out for a few hours.:::::

"I only gots ten bucks to spare," I said.

"That's enough, we'll just play for a couple of bucks."

"I don't know how for play."

"Not a problem. I'll show you. Give me five dice. That's all we need."

I went to the other side of the bar and grabbed the dice, which were right next to the cards, not that any gambling went on here. :::::Yeah right.::::: I handed them over to Bob.

"Okay here's the deal," Bob said, "you get a maximum of three rolls and a four, five, six is an automatic winner, that's Ship's, Captain and Crew. One, two, three is an automatic loser. You can set dice aside and stop in one, two or three rolls. If you don't get four, five, six you save the best dice. You can stop on any roll and the other player has to beat you by getting better dice in the same or less rolls. If you win you take the money and roll first. Got it?"

"So it like Yahtzee?"

"Kind of, let's play. How about for a dollar?"

"Okay"

I started winning at around 8 PM and kept on winning until 10 PM, when the hotel generator extinguished itself and the lights went out.

I don't know if I couldn't lose or if Bob was throwing it somehow, since he probably had the skill and maybe he was looking to help a kid in need. In either case by ten o'clock that night I had won over one thousand dollars Belize, five hundred dollars American. :::::He was somehow "helping you out." It wasn't the first time he played and he wasn't the kind of guy who lost much.:::::

"Good job, Kid," Bob said by the light of the Kerosene lamp which I sparked as the generator extinguished itself. "Are you sure you don't want to go double or nothing one last roll?"

"No Mon, I be good."

"Okay, have fun with that," he said. "You took me good." He walked out the door, into the dark night and down the beach towards his house about one-half mile down.

:::::He didn't seem upset at all did he? Whistled as he left. Must have been doing a good deed for a kid. Trying to help a kid find a way.:::::

As soon as he left I picked up the money and recounted it. It was the most I ever had. What now?

That night I lay awake in the bunk of the hotel's twenty foot sailboat which I slept in when the hotel was full. The water gently slapped the fiberglass hull. I knew I didn't want to stay here anymore. I was no longer attending school at Wesley College in Belize City and that was not an option. I didn't think that moving back down the beach to San Pedro would help. There really weren't any jobs there. I had tried my luck as a fisherman and might be able to do it again, but I didn't want to do it the rest of my life. I broke up with my girlfriend in town and was going out with Susan now and how would I/could I make a future? I came to the realization that my future was not at El Pescador, not on this island, not in Belize, not now and not ever.

:::::Bob probably came to that conclusion before it even crossed your mind.:::::

Around three o'clock that morning I decided that I would take my winnings, go back to Milwaukee and join the military. What else could I do? I was a high school drop-out with no job prospects. I didn't have a job in the United States. I had no job here. I had a girlfriend whom I loved. I was eighteen now. It was time to go and make something of myself.

The next morning my father told me he heard about my winnings and asked me what I was going to do. I told him my plan about going back to Milwaukee, staying with my Oma and joining the military.

He didn't seem displeased and asked when I was going.

I said, "As soon as possible," upon which he promptly gave me the best four words of advice I ever received. They were: "Don't join the Army."

Within forty-eight hours I said good-bye to my family, I think they were happy to see me go, my few friends and Susan, who was now living with her parents after high school. I took the six-hour overnight boat trip, on the *Elsa P*, to Belize City, bought a ticket on Taca Airlines and headed back to the United States.

Two weeks later I was sitting in San Diego at the Naval Recruit Training Center.

Thank you, Mr. Jones for helping me that night. Thanks for your act of kindness. It changed my life. Sometimes small things become bigger things which become even larger. The simple question of, "Steve, do you want to play a game of dice?" while he was sitting in the same seat that Susan once sat in, at the same exact time had changed my life forever.

I should find that seat and bronze it. I sure would like to sit in it now. I needed a four, five, six right now.

The machine stopped spinning, the lights turned off and it fell asleep waiting on the next victim of its lifesaving destructive force. A couple of seconds later I was unbolted for the weekend.

I kept my eyes open the whole time just as I promised myself.

Day 5 - Monday - June 6, 2011

Thank you for the weekend. Even though pretty much all I did was sleep, it was worth it not to have to go into the cancer institute and get locked down.

The weekend without treatments didn't make it any easier to come in today. It probably made it worse. :::::I wonder what would happen if I called in sick. Can you call in sick to a cancer institute when you are going in to get treatment because you are sick? They would probably frown upon that.:::::

Never mind, I'm here. I've been programmed. After a week, I'm getting somewhat used to it. I get up, take a shower, dress, go downstairs and look at food, force myself to drink a protein drink, take a pill, wish I were hungry, curl up in my chair and wait to go. It's not so bad. :::::Liar, it sucks.:::::

I followed Mike into the room.

:::::Oh machine, I missed you over the weekend. I missed the body mask. Nothing better than being held completely immobile for fifteen minutes.:::::

I reclined onto the frigid steel and was dutifully locked in.

"What is the pattern on your scrubs today? Flowers?"

"Lavender, the color of the scrubs is lavender as well. I thought about bringing some in. I like the way they smell. Last weekend was the Lavender Festival in Vida."

"Nice. Wish I could have gone." :::::No sense in blowing his day up by telling him how his scrubs were making me queasy right now.:::::

"How long have you been doing this, Mike?"

"I've been working here for about ten years."

"You must have seen a lot of people in that time."

"Too many. Do you want any music today? Got a couple of people to get to as soon as you are done."

Now he seemed to be in a hurry. Maybe I should lay off the "How many people you have seen button." Maybe he didn't want to get too close to his patients, can't say as I blame him. :::::Or maybe he just had a schedule that he had to stick to. This place is a Swiss watch.:::::

"Dealer's choice on the music. You decide. I'll just lie here and listen. If I don't like it, I'll get up and turn the dial."

Mike gave me his "Yeah Right" look, switched the radio on to a rock and roll station and walked out of the room. Jimi Buffett came on and began to sing *Come Monday* and right on cue, the machine began to hum along with Mr. Buffett.

The dryer drum which surrounded my head began to move slowly and shoot invisible rays into my immobile head and neck. I zoned out as it did its thing.

"Don't worry kids, you are going to love San Pedro," my father said.

"Don't make us move, please don't make us move," I begged.

"We've had this discussion," my father said. "You don't have a vote in this. We are moving to Belize and trust me, you are going to love it. It will be the adventure of a lifetime. I don't want to hear any more complaining or whining."

"Can't I stay with Grandpa? I don't want to go."

"Did you not hear me? We are leaving next week and that's that," he yelled. "You are part of this family and you are going."

"I am not part of this family. You are not my father."

"You are part of this family and you are going."

Three weeks later we arrived at our home site in Ambergris Caye. I arrived separately from my parents and brother and sister but that was another story.

After we got there, it was a month before I left our secluded home site and went to the town of San Pedro, three miles away. Only one structure stood between our prospective hotel and San Pedro at the time and it was way down the beach.

I haven't been to San Pedro for thirty-five years now and I'm sure it has all changed. Last time I checked San Pedro had almost thirty thousand people, more than thirty times as many as when we arrived. Thirty thousand people on a small strip of land. How it worked I had no idea.

When I went to San Pedro for the first time it was through a cut on the island which led to the San Pedro Fishing Cooperative on the back of the island. The back of the island was brown water intermixed with mangroves and little or no wind whatsoever. The temperature difference between the front of the island, where there was almost always trade winds, and the back of the island, which was usually void of any wind, seemed like twenty degrees. We went to the fishing cooperative because it had the only gas pump in town. When we arrived at the cooperative, I jumped off the boat, and it smelled just like you would expect a fishing cooperative, with its rotting fish guts and stagnant air, to smell. STINK, STANK, STUNK. All three, in any order you want. Next to the cooperative were narrow, ratty, broken down, board missing, short piers with outhouses at the end of each. They were used by almost everybody in the town since there was no running water or septic systems at the time. The vast majority of the people did their business at the over water outhouses which teemed with small fish underneath.

At first glance, and even at second glance, San Pedro was part of a third world country. That's not what it became for me.

For me it was paradise and still is. I'm not interested in going there ever again because I'm not interested in the changes. The town and the people live within me just like they once lived. I can go there anytime I want. Once there were about one thousand people where everybody knew everybody. Paradise. Stinky, hot paradise on the back side of town but still paradise.

It was once three sandy streets which were about half a mile each. The streets were named Front, Middle and Back. :::::Surprise.:::::

At one end of San Pedro was Paradise Hotel, and on the other was the elementary school as well as the sand/dirt airport which the Islander airplanes flew into and departed from a couple times of day. Hopefully the arrival/departure numbers equaled one another, but not always.

While the back side of the town and island stunk from rotting mangroves, mucky water and dead fish, the front could not have been more beautiful. As you looked out from the beaches on the front of the island, the water was a foamy blue with dark and light spots that changed as the water changed depth. About a half mile from the shore stood the second longest reef in the world. It touched the surface and the waves broke over it, frothing white. Outside the reef the waves could be thirty feet high and slamming but inside the reef it was almost always completely calm. Rarely were there whitecaps inside the reef.

Along the front of San Pedro was a forty to fifty foot wide beach which was intermittently broken up by piers which stuck out like teeth, some rotten and jagged and some shiny and straight. A few boats were tied up and bobbed along the piers while other boats were dragged up on the beach, their engines in the upright, locked positions. Some small dories were also pulled up onto the sand along the beach, poles sitting in and sticking out beyond the small eight foot long, eighteen inch wide compartments. The dories were waiting for their next occupants to push them in the water, adeptly stand in them and pole along the shallow waters near the shore. They were the first paddleboards.

Directly behind the beach were most of the larger structures of the town, the tallest of which were four stories tall. Most of the larger structures were small hotels with ten to twenty rooms. All were painted predominantly white, most with blue and green painted trim and shutters around their louvered and screened windows. Also along the beachfront were the cemetery, over one hundred years old, and a cement town square, which doubled as a basketball court and was surrounded by bright pastel cement benches with local advertising for bars and other businesses painted on them. Immediately next to the square was the Post Office/Police Station and St. Leo's College, painted in yellow from top to bottom.

Middle and Back Streets consisted of predominantly small homes, mostly twenty by thirty feet, all on stilts to protect them from the ever threatening hurricanes. Each house was painted in white, most with wooden shutters painted in ocean blue and sea green. Attached to each house was a water tank which stored rainwater from the roofs for drinking, showering and cooking needs.

Whenever we went to town I would walk through the streets taking in the sights, sounds, smells and feels. At first when we arrived, I always wore shoes but I soon learned to live as everyone else on the island did, without shoes. It didn't take long for your feet to get thick soles, the final test of which was to put out a burning cigarette with your bare foot or to step on a prickly burr and not even feel it. When I walked through town I savored the sand and dust between my toes.

In town I could almost always hear Radio Belize coming from the open windows of the houses. It was the "Voice of a Caribbean Nation," and carried incessant British radio such as *Porsche Loves Life* and the *UK Top 40*, most songs of which I never heard before or since. Frankly it sucked, but it's pretty much all there was. Occasionally the sounds of Radio Belize were broken up by the sounds of a Mexican radio station with its Mariachi

Music and Radio Soaps. Lastly there were the sounds of people talking in all different decibels to one another, speaking a mixture of English, Creole and Spanish.

Distinctly missing from town were the sounds of TV, there was no TV available in Belize at the time. As far as I know, nobody missed it.

Every time I went to town the smells also hit me. The two smells which I remember the most were the smell of fresh bread from Sefarino Paz's Bakery which reminded me of my grandmother's homemade bread and that of *Rice and Beans with Pig's Tail* (Belize's national meat) cooking for hours over a smoldering coconut husk fire. Even though I am now almost completely void of taste because of damage to my tongue, it doesn't stop me from smelling those long ago smells. :::::Oh yes, give me a slice of that fresh baked bread with butter.:::::

Most importantly I remember the people of the town. Mostly of Mexican descent, there were also those of African descent, Mayans, Guatemalans, Nicaraguans, South Americans, Americans and even a few Europeans.

I thought about that town as the machine whirled slowly over me. There was nothing I didn't love about that town and yet I haven't been back now for over thirty years. I know that for others there was a dark side to San Pedro but to me it is right here in my head, peaceful and tranquil, just like I want it to be.

The machine stopped and so did my trip back to perfection. A tear went down the side of my face. I missed it so. I missed something that was gone and would never come back. I wish I could turn back my clock to sixteen again but those wishes were impossible. I could never turn back time, it kept charging ahead. I looked at every second, never knowing when it would end for me. I prayed it wasn't anytime soon. In the mean time I could visit my island anytime I wanted.

The town in that third world country and its people had changed my entire life.

Mike was now standing over me. "Are you okay?" he asked, seeing the tear on my face.

"I'm fine, something got in my eye and I couldn't move to get it out. It's gone now." I sat up and put my hands on my face for a second before I stood and headed for my locker.

Day 6 - Tuesday - June 7, 2011

:::::Is it Friday yet? Yeah, No. It's just Tuesday, not even close. Just me and you machine, just me and you. Who the hell invented you? Some sadistic genius bastard, I'm sure.:::::

I reclined and got bolted in.

Earlier today, I thought I was doing fine but apparently the nutritionist didn't have the same feeling. For a woman half my size and wearing glasses, she could let a six foot two, two hundred and twenty-five pound guy have it good.

"You haven't been eating, you have lost four pounds in the last week."

"I'm fine, my throat is sore and I'm nauseous when I eat. I just haven't felt like eating."

"I don't care what you feel like, you have to work on getting food into your system. What have you been eating?"

"I've been eating some oatmeal and instant breakfast, some yogurt, some protein drinks. I'm getting in enough. I have some weight to lose."

"Look, we are trying to keep you strong here. We have had this discussion. This is not the time to go on a diet. Do you want to end up with a tube?"

"That's not going down."

"You need to eat more and get more calories in. I understand your throat is getting sore but it's going to get a lot worse before it gets better. You need to eat everything you can now and do it for as long as you can. I am not kidding around here. If you don't take care of yourself and eat more, you are going to end up with a feeding tube. I don't know how many times I've had this discussion, mainly with big tough guys like yourself and they end up with a tube. If you don't want one, you better get with the program."

"Sure." :::::What a ball buster. I'd give her a 5.8 on the 6.0 Olympic scale of ass-chewing.:::::

Susan sat, silently watching me get the butt chewing. She didn't smile. I got the feeling that she let me go for a week, but if I didn't pick it up she would "tell mommy on me" next week.

I knew Celeste was right, but it was the first time that I was being told to eat.

I remember when I was eleven or twelve, listening to a doctor telling me that I needed to lose weight, "Young man you need to lose weight. I want you to lose twenty pounds in the next couple of months." I suppose he would have told me to cut out the junk food, but in the late sixties, early seventies, we didn't have fast food or really have junk food.

I lost the weight then, but it's been a battle forever. Genetics right?

:::::Yeah, that was it - genetics. Genetics also had cancer take the lives of my grandfather and father. No, wait a minute, my father was not my biological father so no genetics there.:::::

Was it genetics that brought me here, unable to move? No, it was bad judgment by a sixteen or seventeen year old that brought me here.

How is it possible that the things I did thirty some years ago could damage me and the one I loved the most? It didn't make any sense to me.

When I was sixteen and seventeen I was essentially on my own. After I ran away from El Pescador, I really never lived with my parents again for more than a short period of time.

When I went to school at Wesley College and lived in the Bellevue Hotel in Belize City, the opportunity to have sex with six or seven women presented itself. I took the opportunity. What teenage boy wouldn't? It was there right in front of me and I didn't say no. :::::I was indestructible back then. What was the worst that could happen?:::::

Here I was with one of the worst things that could happen. The cancer I had was caused by HPV-16. And how did one contact HPV? Through unprotected sex, that's how.

Since I met Susan and we became boyfriend and girlfriend, I have been completely faithful. So before her I had casual sex as a teenager in the 1970's with a few women and I drew the lucky number and contracted HPV-16. Until a few months ago I thought HPV, or herpes, was a punch line to a joke. As in "What's the difference between love and herpes?"

Answer: "Herpes lasts forever." Ha Ha Ha. Not funny now. Apparently herpes does last forever and you might not know you have it for thirty-five years and then it comes out. How does it come out? At the base of your tongue, that's how. And how do you find out? By your neck swelling up because the cancer on the base of your tongue has spread to your lymph nodes.

So here is the result of my careless actions thirty-five years ago. I am now completely incapacitated from the shoulders on up with a damn contraption spinning around me. Here I am praying for my life for something that I did thirty-five years ago. I don't even know who I got it from but I got it and here I am. Thirty-five years ago!!!

BUT THAT WASN'T THE WORST OF IT. NOT EVEN CLOSE. Last night I went on the Internet and looked up my cancer and HPV again. What I found almost put me on the ground. :::::You said you weren't going to go back and look at it anymore, you deserved to get shocked.:::::

About fifteen years ago, Susan got sick with cervical cancer. Guess what, that's how the virus comes out in women.

:::::She had to go through nine hours of surgery and untold pain because of you. Remember how when she came out of surgery she kept pushing the morphine button asking for more pain medication? Remember? You caused it.:::::

Until last night, I didn't know that I could have given her cancer.

Getting a virus thirty-five years ago which gave me cancer was bad enough, but passing on that virus and giving cancer to the one I loved the most in this world was something completely different. How could I have done that to her?

She didn't deserve it. I made my decisions thirty-five years ago when I was young and dumb and you know the rest of that sentence, but how could I have done this to her? She was completely innocent. Completely. She didn't deserve it.

Not only did she not deserve it, I could not take it back nor could I ever make it better or fix it. I can't unring a bell and I can't undo the damage I have done.

Last night, after I found the information, we had a conversation.

"I looked on the Internet and found out that when I probably gave you HPV, I probably caused you to get your cancer as well. I am so sorry," I said, shaking at the knowledge of what I had done.

"I know, I saw that a couple of weeks ago," she said.

"Why didn't you tell me?"

"What good would it have done?"

"Aren't you mad at me? What if I caused you go get cancer?"

"Did you mean to get HPV?"

"No"

"Did you intentionally give me cancer?"

"No"

"Then what good would it have done? How can I be mad at you? You didn't mean to give it to me, you didn't even know you had it."

"My stupidity could have given you a death sentence."

"It didn't."

"If I had known I had HPV I never would have given it to you. I would never intentionally do something like that."

"I know."

"You are handling this so much better than me. I would be pissed. If I were you I would be so mad at me for giving it to you. You should be mad at me for putting myself in the situation to get HPV when I was young. I could have killed you."

"You didn't know. We didn't even know what HPV was back then."

"I swear, I didn't know," I said.

"It's okay," she said.

"No it's not. I am so sorry. I didn't mean to hurt you. I swear."

"I know."

I stood up, said "I Love You," gave Susan a kiss and headed upstairs. I was in shock and exhausted. How could I?

She should have been mad at me. She should have thrown something at me. She should leave me. After all the stuff we've gone through lately she could have left me and I wouldn't blame her.

I am so sorry, I didn't mean to hurt you and cause you such pain.

How could I have given you HPV and cancer? I swear I didn't know.

Please forgive me.

"Wake up dude," Mike said loudly.

I wasn't asleep. My eyes opened and he began to unstrap me.

Day 7 – Wednesday - June 8, 2011

Dr. Baker was his usual upbeat self. For the life of me I don't know how he can do his job. He is the nicest man, but when he walks into the room I see *The Grimm Reaper*, 21st Century style, without the cape and sickle. The highs must be real highs for him but the lows must be terrible lows. What if you were him? Did you get your hopes up or did you just go about your business and insulate yourself from what you were doing?

Did you try to not get close to your patients, knowing that at any time, for many of your patients, a lab test would come in, or you would look down his or her throat and see death looking at him or her and you got to deliver the news? :::::Yummy.:::::

He's been doing it for almost thirty years and is the Head of the Cancer Institute. He must have felt great satisfaction in successes. Did he wonder if he could have done things a different way or done them better? What if he or his doctors/technicians made mistakes? How did you deal with that? How did you deal with a mistake that might kill someone? Did you just look at the statistics to see where you stacked up? What if you aren't up to the averages? Did people ever just become numbers and statistics? Did you just look at what happened and try to learn from the mistake and never repeat it again? The problem was that a mistake or a treatment could lead to a death.

What brought you to this line of work?

He began the weekly ritual of feeling up my neck. :::::Please Lord, don't let it be worse.:::::

"Everything looks okay," he said. "How are you doing?"

"I'm good. My throat is starting to hurt, I'm getting nauseous and I've pretty much lost my taste but I'm happy to be here. It beats the alternative. It's everything you said it would be."

"Okay." He smiled. "Keep hanging in there. It's going to get worse before it gets better, but so far you are doing well. Try to keep your weight up if you can. Keep eating. I'll see you next week."

I walked out with Susan. "That went well," she said.

"Yeah, I'm okay for now. Hopefully, it won't get too bad. I'm getting pretty tired."

"You're fine," she replied, but I sensed some hesitation in her voice.

I cozied up to my buddy. :::::Whoa, you are such a cold bitch today. Couldn't they have heated you up before they had me lie on you? If they put heaters on the cold steel they'd probably heat it up too far and I'd get burned. Didn't need that. You'll heat up in a second.:::::

My mind went elsewhere after the shock of the cold metal. I don't even remember the bolts locking me down A couple of weeks ago, before my daily radiation treatments started, I had asked Dr. Baker if there were any support groups for what I was going through. He referred me to somebody in the counseling office and they told me that there was a weekly group at seven o'clock on Tuesday's.

Last night I went to the group for the first time.

"Group we have a new member today," the certified counselor said. "He is currently going through treatment. Steve, would you like to introduce yourself?"

I looked around the room. It was a standard conference room with a long table and about twenty seats, twelve of which were occupied. I was the only man present. :::::Just like the waiting room outside of the monster.:::::

"I am Steve Wendt, pleasure to meet you. I am a retired Naval Officer who recently moved to Oregon from Hawai'i. I started radiation and chemotherapy treatments last week."

"What kind of cancer do you have?" somebody asked.

"Tongue which spread to my lymph nodes," I said. "I had three surgeries before I got here and now I am going through thirty-five daily radiation treatments and three chemotherapy sessions. Hopefully that will cure my cancer."

"Let's hope so," somebody said, "my husband had all that and then the treatments killed him six months ago."

Another voice came in, "My husband had chemo and radiation as well, and a year after they were done, the cancer spread to his brain and they said they couldn't do anything. Four months later he was dead." She reached down and gently grabbed a pendant which she moved forward and showed to be. "These are the ashes of my husband," she said, showing me the pendant. "They take the ashes and they mix them with glass. That way I can always keep him with me."

I smiled at the woman and said, "That's very nice."

The counselor finally interrupted the impromptu show and tell. "Ladies, let's slow it down a little. Steve, we keep it informal here. Most anybody can talk about anything. Most of the people in the group are not people who have had cancer but relatives of people who had cancer and have passed away. A few are cancer survivors. It's quite a mix and most of us meet once a week. Ladies, would you like to introduce yourselves?"

"I'm a three time cancer survivor," a woman who looked to be in her fifties said. She had a large Band-Aid on the bridge of her nose. "Please excuse the nose, they dug out some cancer from it last week. I'm okay now. Should be all better within a couple of weeks."

The woman next to her introduced herself. "I'm Felicity. My husband died of cancer a couple of months ago. Lung cancer. Never smoked a day in his life. Started coughing one day and six months later he was dead. We used to come to this, together, every week and he's gone now, so I just come alone now. It makes me feel better to see everyone."

"I've been coming here every week for the past three years," another woman said. "My husband used to come with me. He died a year ago, next week. Colon cancer. They thought they had it all gone, but it came back just when we thought everything was good. It wasn't. Now I come and visit my friends and we reminisce every week. I'm sure you will be fine."

She must have been reading my face. It was probably the look of fear on it. The fear of looking around me and knowing just about everyone here knew someone who died from cancer.

I had come here to seek inspiration, not to leave here in desperation. They continued around the room.

"I've been coming here for a couple of months alone," a new voice said. "Well, I shouldn't say alone. My husband died about three months ago, but he is with me always. Just on the way over here I heard his voice say, 'Don't worry Dorothy, I'm okay.'"

I raised my eyebrows.

"He is always with me," she repeated. "He's right here, right now."

Next to her was an empty chair. I didn't ask, but she caught on to what I was thinking. "No, he is not in the chair right now," she said. "I'm not that crazy." Almost everybody in the room laughed a little. It seemed like uncomfortable laughter to me.

I was glad to hear that there were degrees of crazy in the room. I thought I was going crazy before the next woman introduced herself.

"Don't pay attention to any of them," she said. "Most of them come here because their loved ones did not survive, and they need the comfort of friends and someplace to go in the evening. I'm Mary and I had cancer eight years ago, which they cured. I am a survivor, and I am sure you can survive as well. Most people stop coming here once they believe they will survive. Here is what I have to say: Keep fighting. I'm looking at you, and I believe you can make it. Don't let it get you down. They doctors said it's curable right?"

"Yes, they did," I said.

"Then believe them and fight. Every case is different. What happened to almost everyone here is not typical. But what is typical when it comes to cancer? I don't think there's any such thing. Sometimes people make it, and sometimes they do not. There is no rhyme or reason as to the why and as to the how. Why did any of us or the ones we love get cancer? I don't know. I know it scared the hell out of me and that I'm lucky to be here, but I'm not the only one who has survived this long. There are plenty who have. Will you be one of the survivors? Maybe, I don't know. Nobody does. All you can do is come to your treatments every day, trust the doctors, and do what they tell you and then hope and pray that you will be okay and live to fight another day."

I looked around the room. Everybody nodded their heads. She was clearly the most influential person in the room. The counselor didn't say anything.

They continued around the room. There was a mother who had lost her daughter to breast cancer and was now taking care of her two grandchildren who couldn't understand why their mother was no longer with them.

There was a woman who was a miracle. She had pancreatic cancer which had almost spread. She told me the story that when she went to the doctor for an upset stomach, he diagnosed it as an appendicitis which needed immediate surgery, but when they opened her up, it turned out to be cancer which was maybe within a hundredth of an inch of moving into her intestines. Nevertheless, when they sent her home they told her that she needed to "get her house in order."

"So I went home and worked all weekend, as tired as I was, at cleaning my house and making it spotless. I could not comprehend what they were saying to me. I had nobody to talk too and no family. I was naïve to the world. On Monday I went in for a doctor's appointment and the doctor asked me how I was doing. I told him that I followed his instructions and cleaned my house. That's when he leveled with me and let me know that he didn't think I would be here much longer. That was five years ago. According to him I should have been dead long ago. I'm a miracle. That's the good news."

A couple more relatives of those who had lost their lives introduced themselves before all introductions were complete. Introductions took up about forty-five of the sixty minutes allowed for the meeting.

"Well, Steve I think that's everyone," the counselor wrapped it up. "As you can see, we have quite a group here. Diverse to say the least. Do you have anything you would like to talk about?"

I had a lot. Like why am I here? I thought this was for people going through treatment, but instead this was mostly for those whose loved ones died or for those who were very long term survivors. What about those that were going through treatment? I saw them every day. What about guys? What about those with cancer like me? That's what I needed. I needed to talk to somebody who had gone through or was going through what I was going through. Apparently there was nobody like that.

"No, I'm good."

"Does anybody have anything they would like to discuss?" the counselor said. "How is everyone doing?"

The women got into a discussion about baking, quilting and antiquing for the next half an hour. :::::Yippee.:::::

At the end of the session the counselor let us know that there would be no meeting for two weeks and that she hoped I would join them again in a few weeks.

"I hope so as well," I said, knowing damn well that I would never be back. This did more to scare me than to help me.

"Okay, Steve, you are done for another day," Mike's voice said as he came over to unbuckle me.

After last night I could not get out of there fast enough.

Day 8 – Thursday - June 9, 2011

This is starting to wear on me. My throat hurts, I don't want to eat, and my mouth is going dry. One of the side effects of the radiation is that it's killing my salivary glands, so I wake-up dry as the desert. They gave me some mouthwash and lozenges that are supposed to help me with saliva but all they do is make me want to throw up. I am getting my ass kicked. I bet I sleep eighteen hours a day.

:::::Enough whining Steve. Time to get your stuff together and get through this.:::::

Yesterday, I did what I should not have done. I yelled at my wife. For what you say? Because she didn't pull over the car fast enough when I was thirsty.

We are driving along 11th Street in Eugene and I ask her to stop at a convenience store so I can get something to drink since my throat hurts and my mouth is dry. When my mouth gets dry, I have a hard time swallowing. Did you ever try and swallow and you can't? That's the way it is with me now. The more I think about swallowing, the worse it gets. When I don't think about it, either I'm not swallowing or I swallow naturally without a problem, but when swallowing gets in my head it drives me crazy. It's like you want to pull the trigger on swallowing but you can't.

In any case, we are going down the road to somewhere, just to get out since we are finally having a nice day. Sunny and in the 70's, strange weather for Eugene. I am thirsty and I let Susan know, but she doesn't pull over. I ask again when we are approaching another convenience store and she drives right by it. I think she is feeling the pressure of my asking, just like I feel the pressure of not being able to swallow. She passes another store that had something to drink, I blow a gasket.

"Pull the fucking car over at the next convenience store so I can get something to fucking drink. My throat is killing me," I yell, doing no wonders for my throat in the process.

She explained that she didn't see anywhere to stop, to which I respond with, "You passed three fucking places where I could get some water and you didn't stop at any. Just fucking stop at the next place so I can get something to drink. I don't care what it is, I can't swallow and my throat is hurting and dry. I need a fucking drink. There's a convenience store at the next corner. STOP THERE!" :::::Your throat still hurts from that, doesn't it?:::::

She pulls over, I walk out, get something to drink and return to the car still pissed. We haven't talked since then.

Maybe she doesn't understand how much I am hurting. When I ask for a drink I need one now, not later. Or maybe I don't understand how much she is hurting. Probably both.

I think she is flustered and worn down by all this as well. My bitching, moaning and complaining along with my tiredness and glumness are not helping. I need to be better to her. I need to get my shit together and be nicer. After everything, she's the one helping me here, I can't do this without her.

We've been hurting for a long time now. Ever since I left the Navy, even before then. One of the main reasons I retired was to spend more time with her and my children/grandchildren. For the previous twenty-seven years and change I was committed to the Navy and I spent the hours I needed to move ahead. During my last ten years in the Navy, I was in positions of significant responsibility and it was not unusual that I'd work twelve hours a day and then be woken up three or four nights a week to answer questions about what we needed to do for a certain situation. :::::And every night when the phone woke me up I prayed, "Please God let my family be okay, please let Stephanie be okay." I could deal with the Navy stuff and pretty much not bat an eyelid, but the family stuff scared me to death.:::::

About ten years before I retired, after our youngest child Stacy started school, Susan decided that she wanted to be a teacher. I didn't mind. It seemed like a good idea while I was working all those hours, but what I found was that she was committed first to school and then to her job, just as I had been committed to the Navy for all those years.

The last five or six years I was in the Navy she was so busy working as a teacher for sixteen or seventeen hours a day that she didn't have any time for me anymore. She was doing the exact same thing I did all those years. I had done it a lot longer and put her to the side while I chased my career and now I didn't like it that she was doing the same thing.

So I retired thinking that it would change everything. I thought I knew the damage I had done and that's why I retired thinking we could repair what I had caused. :::::No such luck.:::::

Once retired I needed to keep busy, with Susan working monster hours and the kids being all but gone. Only Stacy was left and she was in high school. So I went to school at the University of Hawai'i and majored in English, intending to get a degree and teach. I also worked part-time as a Counselor at the Hawai'i Youth Correctional Facility. I went to bed about ten (a welcome change from when I was in the Navy), and got up between five and six in the morning. After school and work I would normally be home about four or five in the afternoon.

Now I had more time for Susan, but she had become the one who had no time. She was so committed to her students that she couldn't put her work aside. She would leave about seven in the morning, come home about six in the evening, make supper and then get back to her teaching preparations. On weekends she went to work at least one day and, more often than not, she went to the school on both Saturdays and Sundays. Her hours were worse than mine had been and even when I saw her in person, most of the time her spirit wasn't there. It was back at the school or thinking about a student or with our children or grandchildren or with her friends. It was with anyone but me, or so I felt.

I was getting a taste of my own medicine and I didn't like it at all. I reacted just like I was trained - I pushed to try and resolve it.

The more I pushed for time, it seemed like the less she had. I knew theoretically I should have understood, but in reality I did not. She didn't have to work the way she did, I saw other teachers take the time they needed for their families but I also saw that almost all of her teacher friends were divorced or getting divorced.

So I pushed and I pushed and the more I pushed the worse it got. The more I pushed the less she wanted to be with me and the less she wanted to be near me the more frustrated I got and the more frustrated I got the more she didn't want to be near me and then our kids didn't want to be near me and then I got more frustrated and then I was essentially all alone.

So the very thing I wanted when I retired, to spend more time with my wife and kids and grandchildren, became the very thing I couldn't have, because of my frustration and anger over the situation. We spiraled.

She was very successful in her career which made it worse for me. She was "Teacher of the Year" for her school and a leader who volunteered for everything. Even though I went to college and then worked a job, what I wanted most was to be close to my wife, but in my frustration we were not getting closer. I was drifting, never really happy. I had given up one of my loves, the Navy, to try to get closer to the thing I loved the most, my wife and family, and it had backfired big time. :::::You caused it. That's what happens when you are so worried about everything and you lose track of what's important.:::::

If I were Susan I wouldn't want to be with me either. I was not pleasant for her to be with. I felt like she picked everything over me when I felt that I had given up everything to be with her. :::::Too little, too late.::::: It seemed she had moved on and I was fighting a losing battle. I was fighting it in the wrong way, in the only way I knew how, trying to fix it and getting frustrated. The more frustrated I got, the harder I was on her, thinking that would change her and make her understand what she was doing to us. In reality the harder I fought the more I was jamming a wedge into our relationship. The more I pled for us and tried to use my sense of logic the worse it got. About six months before we left Hawai'i we were on the verge of divorce. After thirty-three years I was getting ready to throw in the towel.

The second to last straw was when our youngest daughter Stacy left the house and moved to California at the age of nineteen. At that point Susan and I were alone in the house. I thought it would be the happiest time of our lives, now that the children were gone and I was retired, but it was not. We were alone but the issues didn't change. The more I complained, the more detached she became, the more I complained.

I think the last straw was when I would have lunch and talk with/e-mail female colleagues from the Hawai'i Youth Correctional Facility about our lives. Susan found out and confronted me. The lunches/talks/e-mails really upset her and when she approached me I did not deny them. She said that I was on the road to cheating. I did not cheat on her. I was friends with my colleagues and the majority of people whom I worked with were women. She was very angry and felt as if I betrayed her. At that point we were all but done. :::::You know you shouldn't have done it, she was right. You were wrong. No excuses.:::::

In a final effort to save us, she decided that we needed a change and we, at the urging of one of Susan's old friends, moved to Oregon which I resented, but consented to. I resented it because she took me to a place where I had never been before, forced me to buy a house which I didn't want (right next to her friend), took me away from Hawai'i which I loved, and took me away from two of my three children and my three grandchildren.

I protested, but she said after thirty some years of following me around in the Navy now it was her turn to decide where we went and if I didn't go we were done.

What was I going to do?

I went, but nothing changed at our new home, although Stacy was now living with us again, having moved up from California which was nice.

Susan replaced me with a new set of friends and with my daughter. :::::What do you expect, you aren't great to be around.::::: Anytime I tried to get into the picture she was busy with her friends, our daughter, her quilting, the church, anything but me.

I can't seem to get out of it. No matter how I try, she says the problems we have are all caused by me. I suppose they are. :::::You are in control of yourself.::::: I shouldn't get frustrated and maybe we can salvage this. How long should I wait? When I don't get frustrated for a period of time it doesn't seem to help and eventually I get frustrated.

It is all too convenient and too bad. It's a never ending circle. I get frustrated, I blow it, she says, "This is why I can't get close to you," and then I stop for a while hoping she'll get closer, which she does not and eventually I blow and down the toilet bowl I go.

And next thing you know I am yelling about getting me some water.

How did we get so far down this road? I have to stop, turn this car around and head back to where we came from. Now. I love her and I'm sure she loves me as well.

Here I am getting shot up with radiation, trying to get rid of cancer that is trying to kill me and down deep I am so damaged and Susan is as well by what I have caused, both physically by giving her HPV and cancer, and mentally by me pushing too hard.

:::::She's still here with you isn't she? She loves you. If she didn't she would have shit canned you a long time ago.:::::

Lord, please help me stop this merry-go-round.

Abruptly, the machine stopped whirling around. I was done for the day.

Day 9 – Friday - June 10, 2011

Three, two, one. Lockdown.

I had a better day yesterday afternoon and this morning. Best of all I apologized to Susan for getting upset and she forgave me.

I was able to eat a little and drink a couple of protein drinks. That put somewhere between four and five hundred calories in me. I should be drinking between eight and ten protein drinks per day but I'm not. I think I've dropped about five pounds since I started radiation. I'm sure I'll find out exactly how much I've lost from Judge Celeste during next week's appointment. She doesn't seem to have a problem letting me know.

The effects of the chemo seem to be wearing off a little bit. :::::Must be just about time for some more.::::: I am a little more tired every day but I'm not as nauseous as last week. Maybe I am just getting the routine down.

Today was the last day of Eileen's radiation treatments for her breast cancer. Over the last few weeks we have been courteous with one another. She's married and has two children and five grandchildren but that's about all I know. When you're a patient here I don't think that you get too talkative about what is going on, nor do you get too close to others. :::::You don't let anyone in. You haven't told more than a couple of people outside your family.::::: She was smiling and happy today knowing that this treatment was over but I'm sure she was filled with trepidation. Who knows if it worked? Who knows how long it would work?

Would it work for me? Would I get another miracle in my life? I've had so many. My life was a series of miracles which couldn't be explained through anything else. Was I about to get another miracle, or were they all used up? :::::Cat's get nine. How many do you think you get? You are well over that nine right now.:::::

Since this happened I have asked for so much. I have asked God to save me. I've always believed in God. I read the Bible just about every day. When I was twelve years old my grandmother told me I should read it every day. If my grandmother told me to do it, I did it.

The Bible I have is old and rat-eared. My father and mother gave it to me for Christmas in 1988. My father inscribed the following:

"There are times in your life where this book will give you the comfort and the understanding we are all looking for. When that happens, remember our love and thoughts are with you.

Mom + Dad"

I didn't know what my father believed about the Bible or God before I received that present. We never talked about it. :::::You hardly talked to him about anything, did you?::::: I don't ever remember him going to church other than for weddings or special occasions. That Bible is now probably my most cherished possession. It's been around the world with me, deep underwater, in faraway seas and on far away operations. When I travel, it travels.

Every day now I hold it up tight against my neck, where I had my operation, and pray before I come over for my appointment.

In 1999 and in 2000 my father was diagnosed with leukemia. The nine month impasse between bouts was the happiest time of his life and it was also the most spiritual. The day after my father passed away I met his pastor and learned that my father believed his life was a miracle. I wish I had spoken to my father about all the miracles in his life but it was not meant to be. :::::He would have told you that those nine months were a miracle and to be grateful for any time you get.:::::

Do some of us get more miracles? Do some not get any? Do we all get miracles and just don't know? Do we get miracles every day and just don't know? Do we make our own miracles? Are they divinely inspired or are they just random coincidences? I doubt if they are random. The things I have seen and been through make randomness highly unlikely to me. :::::There is a higher power out there. You know it. You feel it.:::::

Was it a miracle that my biological father ran into my mother and then ran away and never contacted me? I wonder, was it also a miracle for him? How would I have changed his life? How would he have changed mine? I'll never know.

Was it a miracle that my father ran into my mother and married her or was it just a coincidence? How do people get together anyway? Is love just a chemical reaction and something scientists can't yet understand or is it simply destiny, two people randomly running into each other on a random day at a random time in a random place and bang! :::::Sure, right.:::::

I fell asleep until the bolts started coming out. Thank God it was Friday.

Day 10 – Monday - June 13, 2011

"How are we feeling today?" There was new technician in the room. She was Mike's fellow confidant and I'd seen her before but usually I just passed by her as I walked into the treatment room. She normally sat in the room outside the treatment room, staring at two huge computer screens which showed pictures of whatever the contraption they strapped me into was looking at. Next to the screens were a bank of processors, the brains of the outfit.

"I'm okay, I can't believe Monday came so fast. I needed the weekend. How are you?"

"I'm fine," she replied. :::::I'm sure she was; compared to me. Everything is relative.:::::

She placed the restrictor plate over me and began to bolt me in. She was about five foot ten and must have been very pretty under the lab coat, horn-rimmed glasses and puffy hair. I really couldn't understand all the "back to the future" stuff that was happening now. There was a whole group of people, apparently she was one, who wore things from the 50's and early 60's, like BCDs (birth control devices (really horned rim glasses)), and hair-styles from the same period. It was kind of hilarious to me. It's what my mother had worn and how she had looked when I was kid. When I was a kid I considered those glasses and hair styles those of old people and now here they were resurfacing on young people. :::::Oh, Well.:::::

I opened my eyes and she was gone. I daydreamed right through the final stages of lockdown. The machine began to throttle up.

Not only where there people dressing up in 50's and 60's styles now, there were also people who dressed up like they were from the 1970's. They called themselves Hipsters. Really? Skinny jeans, long hair, hip huggers, vinyl-music, record players with huge speakers, Pabst Blue Ribbon Beer. Are you kidding me? They thought the 70's were so cool. I was there. They were not that cool. John Travolta in *Saturday Night Fever* was not cool. *Xanadu* was not cool. KC and the Sunshine Band was not cool. Okay, there were a few cool bands, Aerosmith, AC/DC, Led Zeppelin, Pink Floyd and The Eagles all brought me into adulthood.

And by the way, get your own music. You got Rap. You got Hip Hop. That's yours. Leave my generation's music alone. Embrace yours. Own it or change it. Oh, and stop modifying mine. Almost every "new" song I hear now is just a regurgitation of the music I grew up with. There are a ton of songs now that even steal the melody or words of songs I grew up with and spit it out as new. Maybe there is nothing new. Maybe all the notes have been used up and now we are just down to recycling old stuff into new stuff. Come on, has every original song been sung? Has every original book been written? Have all themes of music - love, loss, dogs, girls, boys - been so overdone that there is nothing left to say?

When I looked at the hipsters, it was like I was looking at a bizarro version of myself in the 70's. Ridiculous. It is strange how people clamor and look back at times past and find something romantic about it. I was there, it wasn't that great. Vinyl is no better than CD's despite what the critics and Neil Young say. If you think it is better, that's just make-believe in your head.

The machine clicked loudly over me and brought me back. Three red lights came on. Seven were green. It shifted two or three inches one way and then two or three the other. :::::Hurry up and do your thing and let me get out of here.::::: I closed my eyes again and let my nemesis continue on its merry way, shooting streams of zoomies. I was living real time Flash Gordon stuff right here.

Last weekend we went to the Eugene Saturday Market for an hour. Talk about a blast from the past. If you ever wanted to trip back to the bad old days all you had to do was go to the Eugene Saturday Market. It covered a two block area in a park right off downtown Eugene and it was, to say the least, entertaining. It was where, a few months ago, I found out that I was the odd man here in Eugene, Oregon. :::::You aren't an odd man out, you are a dinosaur old man.:::::

In my mind I am a regular guy. I spent twenty-eight years in the Navy, I have been married over thirty years, to the same woman, :::::Even if she had four different personalities during that time.::::: we have three kids, three grandchildren, a dog, a cat, a couple of birds. My hair barely touches my ears, I have a regular mustache, no Fu Manchu or Handlebar. I stand about six-two and weigh about two hundred and twenty-five or two hundred and thirty pounds now. I wear mostly blue-jeans, and normally a polo shirt or a colored t-shirt in the summer and plaid long-sleeve shirts in the winter. When I go out, I normally slip on my Navy or Green Bay Packers ballcap. I wear running shoes mostly, although I own a couple of pairs of dress shoes (brown and black).

Before all this shit I had a beer or two now and then, drank a scotch and soda every once in a while, didn't smoke pot or take any other drugs, barbequed in the summer, ate dinner at six pretty much every night, went out to dinner once in a while, woke up about six in the morning and went to bed about ten every night. :::::Now all you want to do is sleep.::::: My wife drives a Jeep Liberty that is a couple of years old and I drive her pass-me-down SUV, which now has over one hundred thousand miles on it. Just regular guy stuff.

When it comes to politics, I think of myself as independent. I mostly vote Republican but have been known to occasionally give a vote to Democrats if they strike me as honest and share my same ideals. The only thing I truly care about is having a representative who has morals. :::::Good luck finding one in today's world.::::: I don't listen or watch either FOX or CNN exclusively, both are ridiculous. My personal rule is that if I watch FOX for sixty minutes, I have to watch CNN for sixty minutes immediately afterward in order to get some balance. Somewhere in the middle lies the truth.

So, I am, in my own mind, just a regular guy and in most of the country, we've lived in six or seven states, I am a regular guy. I am not completely a regular guy in Western Oregon, not so much so in Springfield, less so in Eugene and definitely not a regular guy at the Saturday Market.

The Saturday Market in Eugene. You know the bar scene from *Star Wars*? That is tame compared to the Saturday Market. At its height, from

June through August, it consists of about two hundred booths.

In one booth is the bearded lady, I kid you not, who sells beautiful jewelry. She has the kindest, sweetest voice, always wears a dress, is about sixty years old and has a beard. Well, not a full beard, but most of a beard and I know she must know but it doesn't seem that she cares. As I said, the jewelry is beautiful but when I hear her voice I do my best to avoid her booth because I don't want to stare and I know I am going to. :::::Unenlightened.:::::

Next to her booth is one of the tie-dye booths. Of the two hundred booths, about one hundred sell tie-dye stuff. Those hundred booths all pretty much sell the same thing. Along with their tie-dye for kids, for adults, for dogs, for cats, for you name it, including tie-dye toilet paper which I saw on Saturday, there are always candles and incense for sale. Plus most of them sell rings made out of spoons, heated up and bent around to fit on your finger or fingers or even better, your toe or toes. :::::Don't forget, they will custom fit a spoon to any of your toes. I bet they'd decline if they saw one of your ugly toes.:::::

There are about thirty food booths, from the organic meat store, to the pasties, to the curried up Indian food and food from Nepal, to a ton of tofu and vegetarian as well as vegan booths. My wife enjoys the meat pasties but I won't eat from any of the booths. Not a one looks sanitary and last weekend I avoided the food area because the smells made me nauseous.

In Eugene I'm pretty much sure that a shower is not a daily occurrence for some of its residents. Before I go out and face the day and especially when I go out and see people, I try to make sure that my hair is washed and combed, my nails are semi-clean, I have deodorant on and my clothes don't have any huge holes or stains. This is not a prerequisite in Eugene, doesn't even seem to be a goal for some at the Saturday Market. The worst of the worst, for some reason, appear to be the food vendors at the booths. Almost all have uncovered dreadlocks, most have dirty hands as well as dirt under their nails and I want to scream: "Dude feel free to wash your clothes and your body before you try and sell me food." I'll give them this, the food lines are always long. :::::Maybe you are the weird smelling one, smelling like soap and shampoo and all. It's like they are trapped on a submarine like you used to be. On a submarine you didn't know how bad you, and everyone else, smelled from the stuff onboard until you got off the boat and your wife threw all your clothes in the garage and made you take a shower for an hour before she'd even hug you.:::::

Maybe they are just organic like the market. I swear that almost every booth is "totally organic" and "local." "Local" and "totally organic" seem synonymous with "gouge the customer" to me. If you say "organic" you can double the price and if you say "local organic" you can triple it in Eugene. People will pay it. It's pure genius. Dress like you are destitute, don't shower or shave and mark up the price under the heading of "local organic." They are huge capitalists. :::::Man, you just don't get it do you? Get with the times.:::::

In direct opposition to the price gouging are intermittent people and booths throughout the market expounding the virtues of societies that are not Capitalistic. You get to hear from those telling you that communes are the way to go, that Democracy and Capitalism suck. When I am wearing my Navy Ballcap I usually get to hear how they feel about the United States.

It's not good and it pisses me off, but I don't stop wearing it. :::::You instigate it by wearing the ballcap.:::::

In every corner of the market there are those singing songs, strumming instruments or banging on bongos. Some of them are very good. Most of them are not. Every one of them has some type of receptacle in front of them to receive any money you may want to give, in direct conflict to what they are singing about. Most are singing about how much everything sucks and about how money is the root of all evil while at the same time asking me to give money to them so they can live. Strange brew. Some singers and musicians are so bad I just want to ask them how much money it will cost me for them to stop singing and/or playing.

Usually right next to the "musicians" are the straight up beggars. They all have signs. Nine out of ten of them are apparently "Vets" which I don't buy. Too many times they are "Vietnam Vets" and only in their thirties or forties which doesn't mesh.

For all the people who beg under the guise of being Vets, it ticks me off worse that some "beggars" really are Vets and that we, as a country, are not taking better care of them. No Vet should ever be on the street corner asking for money. We, as a country, owe them more than that.

Most people in the market crowd are dressed with the same apparel that is sold in the market. Tie-dye shirts, pants, hats. Most of their clothes are ripped somehow, mostly for style. I think it's called distressed and most men and women apparently can't afford a comb or a razor. The funniest part for me is the shoes. A lot of the people who go to the market wear shoes, I hesitate to call them that, with toes. You've probably seen them, they are foot coverings which have appendages which you slip your toes into. I don't even know what to say about that. I need my feet to breath and the style here is shoes with toes, which they wear all year round.

The smell of the market is predominantly marijuana, incense and curry. Maybe it's the smell of tie-dye or dreadlocks. Maybe I'm just overly sensitive to it while undergoing chemo.

There is also a crazy overabundance of "service dogs." It seems every other person has one now. When did this happen? Is it only in Oregon? They have little purse dogs here that wear service dog vests. I heard that you can get your dog a service dog vest if the dog calms your nerves. That's crazy. Anytime you go to a restaurant here there are dogs all over the place. So called "service dogs." The Saturday Market is full of "service dogs" and their owners. It is also full of the remnants of service dogs. It's like a minefield out there. I mean come on, we have a dog, he's great and I love him but I don't take him to restaurants and I wouldn't take him to work and even though he calms my nerves, don't all dogs, I can't claim he is a "service dog." And don't you dare question the authenticity of someone with a "service dog" or you will be classified as a jerk for asking. :::::It's a new world Brontosaurus. A new world.:::::

The machine kept whirling around and round.

The market is where I learned that I am the outsider here. When I go with my jeans and with my plaid shirts or straight colored t-shirts I am the odd man out. I'm the oddity that the bearded woman looks at, and probably laughs at. I'm the minority here. Welcome to Eugene where the different have taken over the earth. :::::You are an antique old man. A crusty old salt. Get with the times or get out of the game.:::::

"Okay, Mr. Wendt. You are done for the day. How was the treatment?"

"Pretty much the same as every other day," I replied.

"You seem to be doing well."

"I hope so, this seems to be wearing me down."

"You'll be fine." The last fastener squeaked as she worked to get it undone. "Looks like we need to oil up our fasteners, they must be getting old."

:::::You are so old that it makes things around you get old prematurely.:::::

Day 11 – Tuesday - June 14, 2011

"I can't get any hard food down anymore. Anything other than a drink will get stuck in my throat. This morning I needed to take my pill, the small one, and it felt like I was swallowing a stone, plus the water made me feel like I wanted to throw up."

"You know what they said, you have to keep drinking water," Susan let me know.

"I will. I just can't take anything thick anymore. Yesterday I tried to eat some Greek yogurt and I threw up while it was going down and it went out my nose. Not nice. I guess I'm on protein drinks and Gatorade from here on out. Only about four weeks to go. I'll try to drink six or seven of those protein drinks. The chocolate ones aren't bad, I can still taste the chocolate a little, but Celeste let me know that their taste might change to something not so pleasant. I think she said 'dog doo,' as if she knew what that tasted like."

"I'll get more."

With that our conversation ended and we pulled into the institute parking lot. We got out and walked through the automatic sliding glass doors, for easy wheelchair access, into the waiting area where Susan and I would part ways. I was shocked after we entered and I looked to my left. One of my waiting room shipmates, Joan, was teetering against the entrance of the treatment area. Quickly, her husband got up from his seat, ran over to her and took one of her arms and draped it over his shoulder. She straightened herself and tried to walk but her knees gave out. She hung onto her husband, knees buckled, arm over his shoulder, her head with the ever present red bandana hanging down. He encouraged her. I heard him say, "Common Honey, you only have three more treatments left," but she could go no further. She was out of energy, out of gas.

I had seen her Friday and she didn't look anything like she did now. She looked like her normal self, or the normal self I had come to know. Frail, maybe one hundred and ten pounds, it was hard to tell since the clothes on everyone getting treatment here tended to be loose from weight loss. Back then she still had plenty of life, no hint of give up. We had exchanged pleasantries and she seemed okay but today everything had clearly changed.

I stared and froze right where I was. From my vantage I could see into the treatment area and it was only a couple of seconds before I saw a doctor and a nurse hurrying through the treatment room towards the waiting room entrance. They passed through the entrance and grabbed Joan just as she and her husband were losing their grip on one another. The doctor took her into his arms, her head hanging over his forearm, and took her into the treatment area, her husband following closely behind, where they all promptly disappeared into another room. :::::Shit, is that the way it goes down? One day you are fine and the next.... Who the hell knows?:::::

As I stood there, my knees began to quake. The deck of the ship was rolling as the waves hit. "Let's sit down for a minute," I said to Susan. I composed myself enough to stop the rolling of the ship and we slowly walked over to the disgusting chairs and sat down. I sat there quietly, staring at the double doors, which Joan had just disappeared through. Nobody said a word. We were all frozen. I prayed for my shipmate's well-being as I am sure many others did. After about a minute a nurse came out and called somebody's name as if nothing had happened and it broke the spell. Once the person called got up, everyone started talking again and moving around.

"I'll see you in a few minutes," I said to Susan. I stood up and looked over toward the puzzle table, which had nobody sitting at it, and I contemplated flipping it and watching 1000 pieces of cut up cardboard lavender descend upon the room. I hate lavender. I hate this shit.

"I love you," she replied.

Her words calmed me. "I love you too." I headed out, past the puzzle table, without flipping it, through the treatment room entrance and to my locker, complete with temporary tape. Joan was nowhere to be seen. Was she still in one of the dreaded offices? Did an ambulance come and get her? Maybe she… :::::Maybe anything, you don't know. Nobody knows except those who picked her up and they probably don't know either. Nobody really knows. Ha Ha Ha. The joke is on us.:::::

I changed into my goofy gown and went to the cubicle where we waited for our names to be called. No conversation today. None. One of us was missing and not because her treatment was done. There were only two of the original four women left now. None of us wanted to talk about it. What could we say? We all knew that one false step by our doctors or ourselves, or if our cancer decided to kill us, was all that stood between us and what happened to Joan this morning. Each one of us could disappear just like Joan had. :::::Poof and we are gone.:::::

Fifteen minutes later they strapped me in for my daily rollercoaster ride. The machine started its takeoff sequence and I closed my eyes. I didn't want to see what it was doing to me today. I could feel what it was doing to me, didn't need to see it. Couldn't see it anyway. It was an invisible razor blade and it was destroying my throat and neck. In the last few days I had begun to acquire a wattle. Just like the skin that hangs under a turkey's neck. It was given to me compliments of radiation. The doctor said it would probably shrink but it might also be one of the permanent side effects of the treatments. Nobody knows.

:::::Let me see, I got a wattle, couldn't swallow, lost all or most of my taste buds, a dramatic lack of saliva. I'd take it. At least I got my hair.:::::

I thought about the precarious times I had made it through in the past. It was a wonder I was alive.

Four times I'd been sick and less than one hundred years ago each one of the four times would have killed me. Once I had severe hemorrhaging after my tonsils had been removed when I was a kid, twice I had pneumonia and another time when I got Graves' Disease in my thirties. All four of them were once guaranteed death. That's not even counting this illness which makes five times I would be dead without modern medicine.

:::::But still the doctor's don't know. For every one of those illnesses you still could have died. Every one. The doctors think they have it and the first four times they did, but it's not totally up to them. It's up to so many things.::::

What are the number of times that I'd come close because of bad decisions or fate?

Back in 1973, when I was fifteen, we were all sitting in our twenty by twenty home in Belize as our hotel was being built. At that point the home contained two rooms, a small kerosene stove and refrigerator, two three-high bunk beds in each room and a small toilet area that was not yet hooked up. The only electricity we had at the time was supplied by a small generator which my father had purchased and had recently been wired to the house. We'd start it up for a couple of hours a day.

"Steve, go and fill up the gas tank of the generator so we can have a few more hours of light," my father said.

"Gunthar, don't you think you should do that?" my mother interjected.

"No, he'll be fine. Steve go and do it now, before it gets completely dark. Do it just like I do."

I got up and walked outside, grabbed the gas can, which was under the stilted house and carried it over to the generator which sat inside a recently constructed wooden enclosure. I contemplated turning it off before I filled the gas tank but I had seen my father fill the generator while it was running. He said to do it just like he did and so I did.

Within seconds I had filled the gas tank and the gas ran out from the top of the tank and onto the generator which promptly blew up.

I remember thinking "Oh No," hearing a whoosh and an explosion.

A second or two later I saw my father run out of the house and I looked at him and back over toward the generator and the wooden structure it was surrounded by. The structure and the generator were engulfed in fire.

Somehow I was about thirty feet away and the gas can was about twenty feet to my left, away from the house. I had no idea how I got there. None.

My father ran over to me. "Are you okay?"

"I'm fine." I looked down at my arms and the rest of me. Not a scratch or a burn. Nothing, not a singed hair on my head or anywhere else. I stood up.

My father looked me over. "You look fine," he said. "Why did you fill up the gas tank with the generator running?"

"Because that's the way you do it."

"I do not, I always stop it first so this kind of thing does not happen. Do you know how lucky you are to be alive? The explosion could have killed you. Now we don't have a generator."

"Sorry. It's the way I saw you do it."

"No, it's not. Now we don't have a generator. Now what?"

"I don't know."

We roughed it for the next four months before we got a replacement generator. I was never asked to fill any generator with gas again. I never figured out how I got thirty feet away from it. Maybe I got a running start and didn't realize it, maybe the whoosh blew me away, maybe, maybe, maybe. Maybe a whole bunch of things, definitely something I couldn't understand nor something anybody else could make me understand.

My first job as a runaway was as a lobster fisherman. Not in the conventional sense. In Belize the lobster fishermen did not use lobster pots. They used forty foot sailboats which had ice compartments and carried dories. The sailboats, along with four or five fishermen, sailed about seventy miles from Ambergris Caye to such far away destinations as Turniffe Islands, Half Moon Caye and Glover's Reef. The fishermen would go out for about ten days at a time, just about as long as their catch of lobster tails would last on ice during any given trip.

I had hooked up with a boat which was owned by the brothers of my girlfriend, Mireya. She had threatened her brothers and made them take me fishing. Her brothers were savants when it came to fishing, I was the duty idiot trying to do my best.

One morning about five days into one of our trips, I was teamed up with Bacalao, Mireya's younger brother. We dove for lobster using hooksticks: three foot long, approximately one-inch thick, straight round wooden sticks, which had a large hook securely tied on the end. With those hooksticks we dove the reefs and looked for spiny lobsters. When we found one, we reached into the coral with the hooksticks, hooked the lobster between the tail and the body, drug them out of their crevices, brought them up to our dories, dropped them off and dove back down to look for more.

Bacalao and I, using the large, two-man dory, free dove up and down, back and forth through the reef. We looked and each found a few lobsters throughout the early morning. About half way through the morning and about a mile from the sailboat, I spotted a large turtle and swam towards it. I was surprised that it didn't speed up or protest when I swam up to it and grabbed its shell simultaneously behind its head and at its other end. It was about three feet long and I steered it towards the dory.

When I arrived at the dory, Bacalao came over to help me flip it into the little boat. It was big and heavy, weighed one hundred and fifty or two hundred pounds, but Bacalao and I managed to flip it over belly side up into the dory.

What we saw when we looked at its belly was quite disturbing. It had large fresh bite marks, clearly from a large shark, from one end of its underside shell to the other. Blood was coming out of the bite marks.

"We need for trow dis back in, gets in the dory and gets the hell out of here," Bacalao said. "Dat one big shark. I no want for run into it. Plus der be blood all over dis water now and der is gonna be lots of sharks. Come on, let's trow it back in and get in the dory and head back to da boat and rest for one while."

We threw the turtle out, jumped into the dory and paddled back to the sailboat. Within the hour we were joined by Senon and Ramon, our fellow sailors. Bacalao let them know what was going on and we all ate lunch before we headed back out to get more lobster. Hopefully the water had cleared of blood.

Early in the afternoon, Bacalao and I headed back out to an area of the reef about a mile away. As we got there, Bacalao and I put on our masks and fins and grabbed our hooksticks. Bacalao jumped in just as I finished getting ready to go.

Not a second later, I saw one of the miracles of my life. I distinctly remember Bacalao coming straight out of the water, all the way out, taking two steps on top of the water with his cheap black fins, like a Jesus Lizard, and landing cross legged in the dory, his mask and fins still on and his hookstick still in his hand. His eyes, inside the mask, looked huge and he didn't make a sound. His dark brown skin was now much lighter.

With my mask on, I looked to the area Bacalao had come from and a Hammerhead shark breeched. It was huge, maybe twenty feet. When it breeched the eye on the left side of his hammer looked directly at me. Its eye was dead cold. It looked at me as if to say, "Stay out of my way, this is my fucking ocean, you would be dead if you went first," and then its hammer went down and the rest of the huge shark rolled over the surface and headed back down into the ocean. I have no doubt that if I had jumped into the water first, I would now be gone.

I grabbed a paddle and started paddling back to the boat as fast as I could with my mask and fins still on.

"Bacalao, are you okay?" I asked, paddling frantically.

He didn't say a word. He just sat there like Snorkeling Buddha, with his mask and flippers on and a hookstick in his hand. He was breathing but that was about it.

I kept paddling frantically, afraid that the Hammerhead would surface under the dory, and knock us into the water. Plus this stupid dory was painted dark green, just like a turtle. What if he decides to attack us? These damn Hammerheads are known to be territorial and we were invading his territory. Compared to that shark, the dory was nothing and we were nothing. If we ended up in the water and he wanted to kill us, we were done for.

I looked all around me in terror as I kept paddling for the sailboat. "Please God, save us. Please don't let that monster get us." After I said my prayer, I screamed for Senon.

Bacalao and I arrived at the boat about ten minutes after I started heading over. "Come on Bacalao, get out of da dory and onto da boat," I said.

He did not move. Still Snorkeling Buddha. I kept telling him to get out of the dory. Nothing. Finally after a couple of minutes he said, "Dat one big shark."

Senon arrived in his dory right after Bacalao mumbled his statement and I explained what had happened. Senon and I got out of our dories and each of us grabbed Bacalao by an arm and dragged him onto the boat. It felt like he weighed a ton in the dead weight Snorkeling Buddha position. Right after we got him up on the boat Ramon arrived and I explained what happened. He looked at me skeptically.

Ramon and Senon kept asking Bacalao questions but for the first hour all he said was, "Dat one big shark."

Eventually he started to snap out of it and within three hours he seemed semi-okay. He said all he remembered was jumping into the water, seeing dat big Hammerhead and arriving back at the sailboat. Nothing more.

Even though it was early and we could have done a lot more diving that day we did not. Ramon told Bacalao, Senon and me that he had heard rumors of a big Hammerhead here at Glover's Reef but he didn't think it was a big deal. He was wrong. The next day we sailed for Turniffe, all hands safely onboard.

I will never forget the look on Bacalao's face and how he walked on water. I was not as agile as Bacalao and I never would have gotten out of the water. At best my torso would have gotten out of the water and my legs would have been dangling. I would have been bait. That shark would have killed me.

Later that run, on Turniffe I had another little run in with a shark.

I was alone with a little dory, diving around coral heads in about six feet of water. Round and round I would go, looking for longosta in every nook and cranny of the coral heads. I'd been out for about an hour, moving along and finding a few lobsters, nowhere near as many as the professionals. At one point, I rounded a coral head and looked up. Around the corner from the other direction came a big old bull shark. We looked each other in the eyes and he turned around and swam away. Apparently I had scared him as much as he had scared me.

:::::Liar. He scared you a lot more.:::::

I quickly pulled myself up on the nearest coral head, whose top was only about six inches under the surface of the water, ripping the skin off my knees, making myself bleed, and stood up. The water was up to my ankles and my blood was trickling into it. I started yelling and stood there in my facemask and fins watching my dory float slowly away. I was not getting in the water to retrieve it. Sharks were near and my blood was dripping into their water. I would stand here all day and night if I needed to. I screamed for about fifteen minutes and eventually Bacalao came, picked me up off the coral head and retrieved my dory for me.

I went back to the boat and didn't get into the water for the rest of the day.

Scared as I was and as sympathetic as Ramon, Bacalao and Senon were, I was in the water the next day just as they were. Just business. When you are that age you have no idea how close you came to the end.

After those two incidents, I am slightly afraid whenever I get in the ocean. The Hammerhead made it clear that this was his "fucking ocean" and that he would have gotten me if I had gone first.

I know those sharks put the fear in me. I wonder if Bacalao had any?

How many other miracles had I had? How about on submarines and ships. How many times had I been in precarious situations, fires, flooding, emergencies that could have killed me had it not been for a miracle? Every second on a submarine could be your last second. How many miracles in everyday life had I had that I just didn't even know about?

Are all my miracles up? :::::You are way past nine now, Steve.:::::

"Okay, Steve you can get up now," it was the female technician's voice. It was a lot more pleasant than thinking about those damn sharks.

Day 12 – Wednesday - June 15, 2011

Another day, another dollar, another dose of radiation.

I'm getting to the point now where all I do is get up, shower, try to do something for an hour and then go to the clinic for my dose.

I met with the Weight Police again yesterday after my treatment. It's a broken record. I'm doing the best I can and nobody is cutting into me to put in a tube. The only way they are going to get one in me is if I pass out and they put one in. :::::Sure, tough guy.:::::

Yesterday I tried to start walking around outside on our lanai at 6:30 in the morning, just trying to get some energy and exercise, but when I did it made too much of a ruckus and Susan and Stacy asked me to walk somewhere else since it woke them up.

Today I walked out on the driveway with our dog Kona, round and round we went, for about fifteen minutes. After that, I was done. Before I started all this a few months ago I ran five or six miles a day. Look at me now, fifteen minutes of walking wipes me out.

After my treatment today, I can go home to my Amish chair and curl up with my star-spangled quilt which was made for me by our next door neighbor. It's very nice and she really went out of her way to get it done quickly for me. :::::Probably thought I was going to die soon.::::: I love it, but it's almost too nice to use.

I'm daydreaming today while I spend my time in my machine. I'm not even hearing it click or clack or spin. I can't even see the lights.

The woman who went down yesterday, Joan, was not with us today. Somehow I don't think she will be back. I don't want to ask. I don't want the answer. Some of the possibilities are too hard to take. She was almost done, just a few days of treatments left. I'd rather just ignore it than face it. :::::That's the way to man up. Once upon a time you were tough. Not so tough now, are you?:::::

This morning during my weekly appointment, I spoke to Dr. Baker about the fear associated with cancer. He told me that some patients tell him that it frees them and allows them to stop being afraid of everything.

Okay, I don't get it. I am afraid all day, during every waking moment. My diagnosis didn't free me. It paralyzed me and makes me live in fear.

Perhaps it's my training. I was taught to try to control everything, every minute of every day. I was taught to mitigate the risk and reduce it in every way. For twenty some years I served directly with the Submarine Force. Every day we strove to reduce the risk and increase the safety associated with the operations of nuclear submarines. If we didn't, we would all be dead. :::::You aren't in charge now, are you?:::::

Those submarines are essentially spacecraft. They operate in a world that is totally foreign, in a world that requires you to make your own oxygen, clean your own air, and make your own fresh water for drinking. In that world we are surrounded by salt water almost all the time, the deeper we go the more pressure there is on that hull, the more pressure there is on that hull the more dangerous it is for us. We produce our own power from a nuclear power plant. We sleep next to weapons, potentially big weapons. We live in a world that is totally self-contained and we rely upon ourselves and the engineers that designed those craft to protect us. We are working inside a beer can that can crush at any moment from the pressure around it.

What happens when we don't protect each other or learn and improve on a daily basis is potentially catastrophic. In the 1960's we lost the SCORPION and the THRESHER. All hands were lost on both. Once that hull is breached, or in the case of an explosion, or a problem with the power plant, or any one of a thousand problems, everyone can die - quickly.

More often than not, in the event of a major catastrophe, everyone dies. In World War II, fifty-two U.S. Submarines were lost in the Pacific. In almost all cases, everyone died.

So what do we do? We work to mitigate the problem and be safer every day. For any problems we have, we create a lesson's learned and give it to all submarines so that everyone knows what can happen and what to do to/not to do to prevent problems.

We have thousands upon thousands of pages of instructions and tech manuals which let us know what to do and how to operate all the equipment so we can all survive. We have extensive qualification programs which are strictly adhered to so that we can rely on everyone on the ship to protect one another in the case of emergency.

I was a specialist in the Administrative Field. Every day I lived by procedures. If you used drugs we discharged you. If you had a medical problem you saw a doctor who, based on procedures, would tell us if we could keep you onboard the submarine or not. If you had any problem, we would use the procedures and guidelines and decide how to solve the problem. If there were any new problems, we would make the best decisions we could and would learn from any mistakes to ensure nobody made the same mistake.

Everything was controlled from Alpha to Zulu. We lived by rules and procedures. We lived by those roles and procedures to save our lives and the lives of others. If you broke the rules there could be terrible consequences.

That's how I am trained, to mitigate the risk and do things in an established pattern which prevented catastrophes whenever possible. That's how I tried to live my life, within a given set of parameters.

For me those parameters controlled the fear until now. I always thought if I lived by the established rules and within the established parameters what I could control the fear.

Cancer changes all that. I am faced with a situation I have little or no control over. The doctors provide the parameters but they don't necessarily work. The parameters they set don't fix all the problems. In my case, they don't fix ninety percent of the problems, they don't fix eighty percent, or seventy-five, or seventy. No, statistically they fix sixty-five percent of the problems for five years. If you make it five years you survive. I don't even know where they got that. Why not ten years or why not until you reach your life expectancy. I guess that they had to have some end date to base the statistics on.

I imagine a ship at sea where we only fixed sixty-five percent of the problems and the other thirty-five percent of the problems caused death within five years. That would surely be unacceptable. That could never work. Those ships would never go to sea. That was World War II stuff, where one third of our ships were lost. That was no longer acceptable. We are so technologically superior that I don't think that would ever happen again. But you never know.

Here I was. If three of us were standing in a line, five years from now two of us would be left. One of us would be dead. Those were the statistics.

Somehow that was supposed to remove the fear and to make me free.

That doesn't cut it for me. One third of us dying doesn't do it for me. For almost fifty years we had not lost a submarine because of good procedures and equipment and engineers. That was closer to doing it for me. That could make my fear manageable.

Here I felt as if I were along for the ride. The doctors would do what they did and this machine would do what it was told to do. My body would respond the way it would respond. For the most part I didn't control how my body reacted. It was genetics somewhere in my body that controlled how my body would react or maybe what I ate this morning or consumed for dinner eight weeks ago or maybe what I did thirty some years ago. Who knows? The procedure I was going through did not help me control my fears, nor did it set me free. Knowing I had no control over the situation made it worse, not better. I would have done anything to mitigate the situation but there is not much I can do now.

I want to fight this on my terms and do things under my control to get better but I really can't, other than doing the things the doctors tell me.

:::::You want a set of parameters that guarantee if you do the right thing, everything will be okay and you'll get better. That's not the way it works.:::::

My hands are off the wheel and somebody else, God, I hope and pray, is in charge and wants to let me stay around for a reason.

I just want to be around to live.

Please God, let me live.

Day 13 – Thursday - June 16, 2011

I did not want to be screwed in today.

Last night I had a dream that I died. I was in a coffin, lying down just like I am now. I was strapped into that coffin by the same head and shoulder gear I am currently residing inside of.

At my funeral nobody, except my family, and not all of them, came. I am always so afraid of not doing well enough. I always tried to please others, no matter what, but down deep I am anti-social, I guess.

Didn't I do enough?

My whole life revolved around the Navy from 1976 until 2004. I was engrossed. I had very few friends outside the Navy. I was chasing it so hard that I didn't realize what I left behind as the years ticked by. When we left Hawai'i, I left what friends I had there as well. I was constantly looking ahead rather than cherishing where I was.

In the service we made friendships but they were many times only for three years.

Rarely was I ever stationed anywhere for more than three years. You came to a new duty station and you left three years later. By the time you left a command, everyone who was there when you arrived was gone, since they had already spent their three years there. It was the Woody Hayes offense at Ohio State except instead of three yards and a cloud of dust, it was three years and a cloud of dust. After three years, you picked up stakes and left again to somewhere new. I was stationed at nine different commands in seven different homeports: San Diego, Groton, Bangor, Spokane, Norfolk, Charleston and Pearl Harbor. You moved in and a little while later you moved on.

Although your relationships were close while you were in any given place, they were usually not very deep. As a sailor, you could run into another sailor that you knew twenty years ago and you had a common bond, language and set of experiences that you could hold on to, but there were other things that didn't necessarily come out. Most times relationships in the military were superficial. They were professional and chummy but rarely did you share any inner feelings with anyone. Genuine feelings were too hard to give up and they made you seem weak. You never wanted to appear to be weak.

After three years you would transfer, lose touch, then move on to your next duty, knowing that you could run into old shipmates at any time and renew your relationships as if they had never ended. You always shared the USED-TA-FISH, but that's about it.

If I died, my military friends would quickly shake their heads, say "He was too young," wish me "Fair Winds and Following Seas" and "Sailor, Rest Your Oar" and move ahead. I've served with thousands of men and women and many of them are gone now. You get so used to it. They all affect you, but you move on.

Yesterday afternoon, I looked up one of my old Executive Officers, a mentor, on the Internet to see if we could possibly connect. I needed to talk to someone.

Commander John F. Gabovchik was one of the greatest men I ever knew. I hadn't spoken to him for maybe fifteen years but I still looked up to him. I needed him yesterday.

I was shocked when I Googled his name and out came an obituary. Two weeks ago he died peacefully at home of lung cancer.

He grew up in the Navy just like me. We both enlisted at eighteen. He grew up in Cleveland, Ohio. When he joined he wanted to be a musician, he was a very good trumpet player, but the Navy had no openings for musicians, especially those as smart as he was, so they put him in the Nuclear Power Program.

By the time he was twenty he was a second class petty officer stationed onboard a nuclear submarine. By the age of twenty-eight he was a Chief Petty Officer and went into a program that would let him become an officer. He studied Nuclear Engineering at Vanderbilt University and graduated with honors.

After graduation came the glitch in his career. He was commissioned as an Ensign in the Navy and he wanted to go back to submarines as a Nuclear Power Officer. The great Admiral Rickover wanted him to go to Washington, D.C. and work in the design area. Ensign Gabovchik insisted that he go to a submarine and Admiral Rickover kept on turning him down. Finally, they had a face-to-face and Admiral Rickover told him he was never going to be a Nuclear Power Officer on a submarine and if he wanted to go to submarines he was going to be a Strategic Weapons Officer which did not require the approval of Admiral Rickover.

John F. Gabovchik told him he loved submarines and that he would rather serve onboard a submarine as any type of officer than be in Washington D.C. with a bunch of design guys. And so it came to be that he, although imminently qualified, was rejected from the Officer Nuclear Power Program by Admiral Rickover himself. He went to submarines as a Strategic Weapons Officer which meant that he could never be an Executive Officer or Commanding Officer of a Nuclear Submarine. Every year after he was initially rejected he diligently applied for the Nuclear Power Program and every year he received a personal note from Admiral Rickover letting him know that he would NEVER be in the Nuclear Power Program again. Despite Admiral Rickover's disapproval, Commander Gabovchik served admirably for a couple of tours onboard submarines as a non-nuclear officer. He was never allowed to be a Commanding Officer on a submarine because of his rejection from the Nuclear Power Program.

He also had a great tour in England as a Naval Attaché. He spent a few years there with his wife Martha and their son Mitchell, who both meant the world to him. After his tour in England, he reported to the USS L.Y. SPEAR as the Executive Officer.

Onboard the SPEAR, I was given the privilege of getting to know him. His given name was John F. Gabovchik, but he was "XO" to me. By the time we met in 1989, he was forty-nine years old and he smoked like a chimney. It seemed there was never a time when he didn't have a cigarette, or two, lit in his ashtray. He was kind and friendly and going bald, worked about twenty hours a day, stayed on the ship rather than go home more often than not, and always took care of the people who worked for him.

I had reported to the ship about a year before his arrival. That year was known to me as the *Reign of Terror* onboard the SPEAR. We had a Captain who was a screamer and lived to drive us all crazy. The Captain was unique to say the least. The Captain was about five feet six inches tall and one of his quirks was that the taller you were the more he hated you. I am over six feet, so he hated me more than most.

I got to know the XO two days after his arrival.

"Ensign Wendt, you are a fucking idiot," Captain Terry said. "Why can't I get you to do anything right? All I want is to get the correct number of people onboard. Right now we are one hundred people short of the sixteen hundred people we need onboard."

"Sir, that means we are above ninety percent, which, according to the Submarine Force Atlantic is excellent. We have the best manning of any tender in the fleet," I replied.

"I don't give a fuck. You are failing if we aren't at one hundred percent."

"Sir, we are never going to get to one hundred percent, no surface ship ever does. This is not a submarine, it's a surface ship and we won't get there. I know we can do better, but realistically we are about as good as we are going to get with the overall manning problems in the Navy."

"Are you fucking deaf?" he said

"No, Sir," I said

A new voice from the door chimed in. "Captain, can I talk to you for a few minutes alone? It's very important." It was the XO.

"When I'm done with this idiot," the Captain said.

"Now Sir. It's important. Ensign Wendt, please wait outside."

I sat there, waiting for the Captain to blow, not knowing if I should move. The Captain looked at me. "Get out of here. Wait outside," he said.

I stood and did as told, walking past the XO, who was about on inch taller than I was. I thought to myself, *The Captain has a new target.*

The XO stepped into the Captain's stateroom and closed the door behind him. I stood outside the stateroom waiting.

"What's so important that I can't counsel that idiot?" I heard the Captain say through the door.

"He is not an idiot," the XO said. "You know he was a Leading Yeoman on the first Trident Submarine and he's not your typical Ensign. He has twelve years of service. Your counseling style isn't going to work with him. He knows what he is doing, he spends about twenty hours a day here trying to do a good job. Everyone I talked too says he works hard and is making things better around here. You need to pull back a little."

"All you guys who were ex-enlisted are the same," he said. "You guys think you know everything and you always stick up for each other."

"We are not all the same, but maybe you should consider that ninety percent of the officers onboard this tender were ex-enlisted, most have more than ten years of service and all of them were selected based on their proven abilities rather than on just having a college degree."

"Wendt is a moron."

"He is not. Give me a chance to work with him and lay off him and all the other officers. You have been getting things done by screaming all the time. Your officers don't respect you, they are only afraid of you."

"I don't give a fuck what they are, as long as the job gets done. Let them be afraid. Maybe they will work harder. Get the fuck out of here XO, and send that moron back in, I'm not finished with him."

"No, I'll get the fuck out but I'm not sending him back in."

"I'll shitcan you if you don't."

"Go ahead, but how's it going to look that you have canned two XO's within a month? Just let me start working with the officers and the crew. Trust me. You will see."

"Get out of here and shut the door behind you. Take him with you."

The XO came out and said, "Come on Ensign, follow me."

We went back to his stateroom and discussed what I needed to do. Essentially he told me "to always come to him first, to always be honest, and to always let him know if there were any problems coming up."

"Thank you Sir, for what you said."

"Just call me XO. I know you work hard and do the best you can. You can do this thing. You are the Admin Officer and I'm the XO. We need to work together to get things done the right way. I know you know the right way. I see you taking care of your people. Keep doing things the right way and we will get through this. Come see me at 1600."

And thus the *Reign of Terror* ended for me. Commander Gabovchik always took care of me and I did my best to take care of him. Where we perfect together? No. Did we always see eye-to-eye? No. Did I see him almost every day at 1600? Yes.

When the ship was in Annapolis and Susan was about to give birth to Stacy, did he send me home? Yes, even though she didn't give birth until after the ship was back in Norfolk.

A few months after the XO arrived, Captain Terry departed and a new CO arrived. Captain Elliott was the best and he let us work to achieve great things for our submarines without screaming.

The two years I was assigned with Commander Gabovchik I learned how to be a Naval Officer. When I became an Executive Officer and Chief of Staff, I emulated him in every way that I could. Not only was he a mentor, he was like a father to me.

On one occasion he even introduced me to his personal friend, Tom Clancy who was visiting the ship at 1600 on a Friday afternoon, after almost everyone had gone home for the day.

Mr. Clancy told me about meeting the XO in England. It seemed strange to me that Mr. Clancy, an insurance salesman, had written a book about submarines and here I knew a submarine officer who was his close, personal friend. I also wondered about the scenes in his books from London. I think they were written about the same time the XO was stationed there. Mr. Clancy was just a "regular" guy who happened to know a hell of a lot about the Navy. :::::Sure he was.::::: He visited the XO on a few occasions during the two years we were stationed together.

Despite our closeness and our working together all day, every day, once I transferred I saw him only one more time and when I did the magic spell was broken. For him and for me. We shared pleasantries but that was about it. Sad.

Yesterday evening I was so distraught that I needed somebody to talk to. My father was gone, I really didn't have any friends I wanted to share my feelings with and I was already being too much of a burden on my family. They didn't need me to continue to drag them down.

Yesterday was too late. I know he would have been there. Why hadn't I told him how much I appreciated him and how much he had taught me over the years? Why didn't I call earlier and tell him how much I used what he taught me every day. He reinforced what I had learned prior to meeting him and he taught me how to become a Naval Officer. Even more than that, he taught me how to stand-up and be a better man.

I am forever indebted to him for everything he gave me and now I can't even reach out and actually talk to him. I missed my opportunity while my life played out. I hope he can hear me now, wherever he is. Thanks XO for all that you did for me.

Have I done enough? Have I fulfilled the example that John F. Gabovchik set for me? Did I take care of others as well as I should have?

I hope so.

"Okay Steve, you are free again. See you tomorrow."

I stood up and shook off the dream. After all, it was just a dream right?

Day 14 - Friday – June 17, 2011

"That's great Steve, you hit your spots dead on. Are you ready for the weekend? Doing anything?" Mister My-Brown-Scrubs-Have-Pictures-of-Sharks-All-Over-Them inquired, angling for some type of response, probably to catch my mood.

I wasn't biting, but I would nibble. "I'll probably spend the weekend sleeping this off. Maybe spending some time outside, enjoying the heat. Plus tomorrow is my wedding anniversary. Thirty-four years."

"Thirty-four years – that's a long time. Are you going to celebrate?"

"Don't think so, I'm kind of not up to it right now."

"That's understandable. Stay still," he said as he headed out. A big Hammerhead shark on his back looked at me. :::::Whatever.:::::

Man, we were so young when we got married. So very young. Susan and I were just eighteen years old. Now look at me. :::::That's right, look at you.:::::

After this treatment I get two days off. Thank you very much. It feels like I've had the flu for three weeks now.

Yesterday I watched ESPN for a few minutes and they were having a discussion about the returning Super Bowl Champions. The Green Bay Packers.

Immediately I went back in time to growing up in Wisconsin in the 1960's.

If you were a kid growing up in Wisconsin in the 1960's you were a Green Bay Packers Fan.

That time was so different from today. We lived on Plainview Parkway in Sussex, Wisconsin, a suburb of Milwaukee. W222 N8179 to be specific. All the homes in the subdivision were about the same. Three bedrooms, one and one-half baths on an acre of land. They were all made of Lannon Stone from a quarry less than five miles away. The homes were twelve to thirteen hundred square feet and we thought we had plenty of room. Every house also had a one car garage, never two. After all, you didn't need a two car garage because nobody had two cars. Didn't need two cars when everybody in the neighborhood had fathers that worked and mothers that stayed home every day.

We also had no cable and TV wasn't something that we watched all day, every day. I remember the excitement when we got a color TV in the mid-60's. First in the neighborhood. Before that we had black and white sets, some with a ridiculous sheet of plastic colored green on the bottom and blue on top that could be placed over the tube. The green simulated the color of the grass and the blue simulated the color of the sky. The reception was through rabbit ears on top of the TV. You got three network stations, ABC, NBC and CBS and a UHF station or two, good for watching wresting with The Bruiser, The Crusher, Doctor X and Verne Gagne on Sunday mornings right after *Gumby* and *Davey and Goliath.* :::::Oh, Davey! Shut up, Goliath!:::::

As kids when we weren't at school all we did was play. In the summer, right after breakfast, I headed out on my three speed Raleigh bike, with my baseball glove hanging on the handle bars, to meet with the other boys in the neighborhood. We would play baseball until one or two in the afternoon, after which we would jump in one of the above ground pools that people had or make our way via bike to the flooded out quarry about three miles away to swim for an hour or two. By three or four in the afternoon we were back playing baseball until dinner time. None of us had watches, so dinner time was when our mothers called. After dinner we headed out again until it was dark and our mothers once again yelled for us to come home.

During the school year, we would play football, basketball or hockey after school every day.

On Saturdays we also played organized sports at the Ball Field in Lannon, a little ways from the quarry. During the summer we played baseball, starting in the Dew Drop League and moving up to Rain Drops, hoping to someday make the Puddles in high school and maybe even to the Lakers, a semi-professional team, after high school. In the fall, the Lannon Baseball Field was converted into a couple of football fields for flag football.

Every Saturday in the fall, hundreds of grade school kids would converge on the fields to play flag football. All of us, except maybe one or two, wore our Green Bay Packers Rawlings Helmets. The odd kids out were the one or two that were wearing Chicago Bears Helmets. Losers. What kind of parents would send their kids out into a sea of three hundred Green Bay Packers loving kids wearing Chicago Bears Helmets? Are you kidding me? They were the complete loners. Nobody talked to them and nobody wanted them on their teams.

Those days of just living and playing were some of the best in my life. I didn't have a care in the world. It was before girls, before high school, before Belize, before I found out that my father was not my father. I was a kid living a regular life in a regular place, day after day in a place without any troubles that I remember.

In Wisconsin, in the 1960's you were a Packers Fan and you were a Vince Lombardi Fan. The first book I ever read from start to finish was *Instant Replay* by Jerry Kramer (No. 64, Offensive Guard) and Dick Schaap. I was ten and I couldn't put it down. I was such a big fan of the Packers that I still have, among my treasured possessions, autographs of Lionel Aldridge and Willie Davis from the 1960s.

The Packers were not just a team and Vince Lombardi was not just a coach. They were a way of life. Vince Lombardi was more than a coach, he was a philosopher. He lived by a set of morals and values that we all tried to emulate. He believed in teams, in family, in God.

I know it's ridiculous now but it wasn't ridiculous then. It's still not ridiculous to me. It seemed so much simpler back then.

You lived your life by a set of rules. You lived your life by Vince Lombardi. You tried to do the right thing. You believed in this country, you believed in everything this country was about.

My whole life I have tried to live up to the following:

After all the cheers have died down and the stadium is empty, after the headlines have been written, and after you are back in the quiet of your room and the championship ring has been placed on the dresser and after all the pomp and fanfare have faded, the enduring thing that is left is the dedication to doing with our lives the very best we can to make the world a better place in which to live. *Vince Lombardi*

Suddenly the machine stopped around me and a couple of seconds later Mike came in. "Steve we are going to have to readjust your mold. It seems that with all the weight you've lost, I need to tighten this puppy up around you. Let me check." He came up around me and retightened the bolts. "Okay, that's better. Hang in there." He exited the room.

:::::Like I have a choice.::::: Man, now the mold is getting loose from all the weight I've lost. I'm sure by next Tuesday I'll be hearing it from my personal weight loss consultant.

The machine started up again and I just watched it go round and round with Vince Lombardi quotes bouncing around in my head.

What has happened to this world since then? Do I still have a purpose in life? Would it be better if I weren't here? Would anybody care? Am I just an old guy hanging on to what I have for no good reason?

Have I done enough? Is the game over? Do I have more to give?

Am I what we used to call a FLOB in the Navy? A Free Loading Oxygen Breather? Do I have a purpose? Am I still worth it?

Day 15 – Monday – June 20, 2011

"How was your weekend?" Mike asked me cheerily.

"Just ducky, I slept through it all. Don't even know where it went."

"Did you do anything special for your anniversary?"

"Told my wife I loved her, that's about all I got in me right now."

"Three weeks down right?"

"Yep three weeks down and four more to go. Yeah!!"

"I'm going to turn on the radio for you listening enjoyment."

He was way too happy for a Monday. "Go for it," I spoke quietly through the immovable mesh. "It'll help time go by while the wheels on this bus go round and round."

"Let's try a little classic rock." He changed the tuner over to 105.5 – FM.

The usual morning shtick was on as the machine began to warm up. Eventually they played a song. Bob Seger came on singing *Like a Rock.*

Like a rock.

THE LOOKING MASK

Once upon a time I was a rock. I drifted back to 1974, I was sixteen.

"Get up!" my father yelled.

"I tired, let me sleep a little longer Mon," I said

"Get up now, you have work to do. We have cement to mix."

"I be up in a few minutes. Just a little longer."

"Now. It's already eight o'clock. If you wouldn't stay out so late with that black girlfriend of yours, you could do your work."

"Leaves me alone." I opened my eyes and saw his angry face glaring down at me.

He reached down and grabbed me. "NOW, I said. You are going out with that black whore and it is ruining your life." His jaws clinched and his face turned red.

I was up now. Our eyes were at the same level and those comments were not going to stand. "Fuck you. She not one black whore." I pushed him and he tripped over the bed, landing next to a spear gun.

As he reached for the spear gun, I bolted out the door and ran for town. I ran for the only peace in my life. I ran away from the hotel and my family. I ran toward her with only the clothes on my back and I didn't look back for months.

Once I got there, my girlfriend got me an eight by ten room with her Aunt for twenty dollars a month, lent me some money to buy a toothbrush and some food, and I began working with her brothers on their lobster boat.

I was sixteen, I had no money and I stood proud. I did what I felt was right. I was in charge of myself, nobody could tell me what to do. I had nothing but I had everything.

I took the verbal taunts from my father, my mother, Mireya's brothers and anybody who called me stupid for leaving a situation where I had everything, but I didn't care.

Where had it gone?

Like a rock.

"Attention," the Company Commander said.

All eighty of us in Company 253 at the San Diego Naval Recruit Training Center on 15 December 1976 snapped to. We stood in formation, ten rows of eight per row. I was in the third row, second from the left. We had just marched onto the grinder for the graduation ceremony. I had joined the Navy in September and here I was at the boot camp graduation ceremony.

"Parade Rest"

Our right feet came out and our hands went to our lower backs in the precise unison which could only be had after eight weeks of training and of living together every day, all day. We were good, we did everything together. We got up in the morning at 6 AM, went to bed at 10 PM and in-between we trained, smoked, joked, took tests, did physical training and studied.

Collectively we acted as one, just as the Navy had designed. They broke us down, then brought us back up and taught us everything they felt we needed to know to start the journey. Physically, I would probably never be stronger. When you are eighteen and they have you do physical training every day, everyone starts to mold into the same body. The fat guys got skinnier and the skinny guys gained weight and got cut. The medium guys sort of stayed that way.

We listened to the obligatory graduation ceremony speeches and went up and down, up and down, attention to parade rest, to attention, to parade rest about twenty times before the speeches finally ended and we marched off.

I was never more ready to restart my life. I stood like a rock, ready to take on the waves.

Like a rock.

In June 1977, I got married to Susan in Southampton, New York. I made two hundred and fifty-three dollars every pay day. Five hundred and six dollars a month, and our rent was one hundred and seventy-four dollars a month. We had the time of our lives. I was stationed on the USS DANIEL WEBSTER (SSBN 626) (GOLD), a strategic missile submarine. On November 25th of that year, while we were visiting Southampton for Thanksgiving, Susan gave birth to Stephanie. The doctor asked me if I wanted to witness the birth, I said no. Back in those days you went to the father's waiting room and smoked cigarettes. After Stephanie's birth, times were a little harder but we still made it with a couple of bucks to spare. We were both nineteen when Steph was born.

I stood up iron straight as the submarine rolled. The Captain approached me along with Chief Bainbridge. They stopped in front of me and the XO read:

"As of the 25th of February in the year 1978, I hereby declare that having completed all requirements and having been examined by a board of his peers, Seaman Wendt is hereby designated as "Qualified in Submarines" and is due all the benefits of his qualification."

We were on a Deterrent Patrol in the middle of the Atlantic Ocean somewhere, on a Strategic Missile Submarine, punching slow holes in the water, keeping the world safe for democracy. The sixty or so shipmates that surrounded me all clapped and the Captain and Chief Bainbridge pinned my dolphins onto the pocket of my poopy suit, shook my hand and walked off.

Their walking off signaled everyone else to come up and shake my hand as well. Unfortunately, when you got your dolphins, you also got them "pinned on" which meant that people would punch your dolphins into your chest. It hurt, but it signaled your acceptance into the brotherhood.

It was the culmination of a year of hard work.

In 1979, I was selected for the pre-commissioning crew of the first Trident Submarine, USS OHIO. When she got commissioned in 1981, I was the leading yeoman onboard as a second class petty officer.

"Petty Officer Wendt."

I looked up. I was sitting in the Ship's Office of the OHIO and the Captain had walked up to my door. "Yes Sir."

"Congratulations, you are a father again. Your wife gave birth to a son a couple of days ago on 2 December. That's great news."

"Thank you very much Sir." I smiled.

So my son Stephen was born and I was at sea, not an uncommon occurrence if you were in the Navy at that time. In the words of one of my shipmates, "Just be thankful you were there for the important part."

In 1985, I heard the words, "You are now advanced to Chief Petty Officer in the United States Navy."

In 1988, I heard the words, "You are now commissioned as an Ensign in the United States Navy."

In September 1990 I was stationed onboard the USS L.Y. SPEAR and I was the Duty Officer.

"Steve," Lieutenant Don Cyzelsky said, "we are having a department party this afternoon. Can I drink safely?"

"Sure, why not?"

"You're the Command Duty Officer and I know that your wife is due any day now. Hell, we sent you home from Annapolis last week so she could give birth, but that was a no go. Are you sure she isn't going to have the baby today? It's 1500 and I'm getting ready to leave. I won't drink if you think she is going to have the baby today. I don't want you to be stuck on the ship while she gives birth."

"I just talked to her and she said she is not having the baby today."

Two hours later I got a call from Susan saying that she was on her way to the hospital to give birth to our third child. Figured.

I called Lieutenant Cyzelsky at the party. "Don't tell me, your wife is giving birth now," he said.

"Yep."

"Good thing I didn't drink. I knew it was going to happen today. I'll be there in twenty minutes."

Don showed up fifteen minutes later and took responsibility of the ship for me ten minutes after that. I headed off to the birth of my daughter Stacy.

Twenty minutes after I arrived at the hospital, Stacy was born on the 21st of September 1990. For the first time I was able to witness the birth of one of my children. It was a great day.

We now had three wonderful children, Stephanie, Stephen and Stacy. We were financially doing okay and we were a family even if I was working sixteen hours a day.

Like a rock.

In 1994 I transferred to the Submarine Force Pacific to be the Executive Officer. I was a Lieutenant. By 1999, I was a Lieutenant Commander and the Executive Officer of the Naval Submarine Support Command in Pearl Harbor.

Part of the deal of being an XO is you always have to be on call. I received calls almost every day and every night, there was no rest for the wicked. I rarely got more than five hours of sleep a night. Not a problem. :::::Yeah right, except for the part that every time you got a phone call in the middle of the night you automatically worried for Stephanie's life. You still hate phone calls in the middle of the night. Nothing good happens after midnight.:::::

Still a rock.

In 2002, I had twenty-six years in the Navy and I was wearing out. Too many nights being woken up at 2 AM.

I decided to get out, but they promoted me one last time and kept me in Hawai'i. I was ordered to the Special Operations Command Pacific at Camp Smith on Oahu and it was not any fun for me.

For the first time I was working with the other armed forces and after having spent all my career within the Submarine Force, it was different to say the least. The other services were downright puzzling to me. They thought different, they moved different.

They Army. I don't even know what to say about them. I was used to the Submarine Force where we skimmed off the upper ten percent of individuals from the Navy. The Army had everything from guys with doctorates to guys who, let's just say, were the opposite. :::::Those guys were like you when you joined as a high school dropout. You did okay.::::: How they operated I didn't understand.

The Marines. I could understand them. They were part of the Navy and worked for the Department of the Navy. They thought almost the same way as the Navy did, but they were the real warfare end of the Navy. As they said, "We love you Navy guys, you give us a ride wherever we need to go and you drop us off when we need to fight." How true.

The Air Force. The Chair Force, the Air Farce. They were the strangest of the bunch to me. Their service only really came into being after World War II when they broke off from the Army. They were a hybrid, part Army and part "New Service." When I talked with them it was strange. I was used to a whole way of life in the Navy. We had our own language, we had our own traditions, we essentially had our own culture. I don't know what the Air Force wanted to be. Their Ho Chi Min hats were strange at best and their talking to each other on a first name basis was mystifying as well. They thought their ways were professional. I thought that their lack of presence, lack of traditions, and lack of command structure were off-kilter. :::::You were just getting old.:::::

When I got to the Special Operations Command it was a mish-mash of all the Services with a Special Operations identity. Special Operators had their own hierarchy. At the top were the Navy Seals, next were the Green Berets and the Air Force PJs, followed by the Army Rangers and Marines, who considered every Marine a Special Operator. Throw in a few pilots and intel guys and there you had it.

:::::Then there was you, a submarine admin guy in a special operations world. Talk about a fish out of water.:::::

I was the J1, Director of Administration/Personnel and Manpower, and responsible for Special Operations Administration throughout the Pacific Theatre. Of the eight Directorates, I worked in the only one run by a Navy guy, me. The Commander of the outfit was an Air Force General.

My whole time at Special Operations Command Pacific the only thing I could do was shake my head. Everything was so off-kilter. It was not that I didn't get along with others at the command, it was like we were talking different languages. I didn't understand them and they didn't understand me. When I said "deck", or "overhead", or "bulkhead", or "head", or "scuttlebutt", or "skimmer", or "bubblehead", they looked at me like I was insane.

I think when I heard the Army Chief of Staff say, "Those fucking Navy guys, I don't understand them," it dawned on me that this Joint Services thing was crazy. All the services spoke their own language and after twenty-seven years of speaking a certain language it was difficult to learn three other languages simultaneously.

Plus I HATED WEARING GREEN. It was probably from my father saying those immortal words to me, "Don't join the Army."

When I was at SOCPAC I was required to wear Seabee fatigues. If I wanted to be a Seabee I would have joined the Seabees. I was a qualified Surface Warfare Officer as well as being qualified in Submarines, I wasn't really interested in dressing like a tree.

In 2004 I decided to retire. Between the work and the stress of home, I was all funned out.

I was not the rock I once was.

In 2004, I began going to the University of Hawai'i where I received a degree in English in 2008. When I started there I thought I was going to be an English Teacher but I found out during my semester of student teaching that teaching in high school wasn't for me.

I'm not sure if I wasn't good at teaching or if I just didn't fit in with the teachers of today. I think I would have made a good teacher but I soon found out that my beliefs and those of many in the teaching profession differed. I was more about the rules and regulations, they were more about the touchy-feely.

In the end, I think my biggest deficiency was that I never really went to high school. I had no pool of information to draw from. Everybody else I went to college with, who wanted to be a teacher, had a relatively recent set of experiences in high school from which to draw from, whereas I had none.

In 2007 I changed my major from Secondary Education to English.

After thirty years the rock was getting worn out.

While I was going to college, I was also a counselor for a non-profit in Hawai'i at the Hawai'i Youth Correctional Facility. I was very successful, but it took a toll on me. Every day I would go into the Correctional Facility, make that a jail, and talk to three or four young men individually or groups of ten to fifteen young men. During the four years I worked there, I saw the depths of despair. I talked to young men who were murderers, rapists, thieves, drug dealers and drug users. I did my best to help them do better. Some would never get out of jail, others would go back to jail over and over and over again. Thankfully, some would do their time and never go back to jail again. I taught cognitive restructuring.

I did my best to get rid of their "stinking thinking" by teaching them how to make good decisions instead of repeating some of the ones they had made in the past. I think I helped some of them, if they wanted to be helped. If they didn't, it was tough. I, however, was always there and always talked to them.

I think half the battle for me, and for them, was that most, or all, the adults in their lives left them or betrayed them in some way. I did my best to be a steadying force for every young man and tried to set a good example while I was there. Most times I would never know if I helped, some of the things we talked about might never sink in, some might not sink in for twenty years and then the light might click on and they would say, "Who was that haole guy, who tried to teach me to make good decisions? Now I get him." Most probably wouldn't remember my name, but hopefully they would snap out of their bad decision making someday.

I also taught groups with partner counselors during that period. I went through seven partner counselors in my four years at the correctional facility. One, a former football player at the University of Hawai'i, lasted for one day. Another, who is an actor on TV now, lasted a week. Those youth could wear you out quick. You went in there with the best intentions and they would push your every button. I was called a "fucking haole" weekly if not daily. After four years I was worn out and in 2009 I left the non-profit.

The waves kept rolling in and the rock was fading away.

I went back to Submarine Force Pacific as a contractor. Once upon a time I had been the Executive Officer there…

"Okay Steve, we are done for the day." Michael startled me to consciousness.

"You might be done with me, but I get my second dose of chemo today."

He unscrewed me. "You'll be fine."

Maybe, but I know this, I wasn't the rock I used to be. My foundation was cracked. How was I ever going to keep going and get through this without my house falling apart? How much more of this could I take before my rock turned into sand and I disintegrated with it?

Too many waves, too much time.

Day 16 – Tuesday - June 21, 2011

Hope. That's what I had now.

Yesterday, I received a gift from one of Susan's friends, Jenn. She sent me an ornament, which was in the shape of an Angel. On it were inscribed the words - Faith, Strength and Hope.

Before I was able to receive the gift from Jenn, I received the gift of chemotherapy for the second time. It least this time I knew what to expect. After radiation I trudged on up to chemo with Susan, headed in and took my medicine. :::::You mean poison.:::::

The room was the same, it looked like the same people, even though I knew they weren't. I was one of the few in the room who still had my hair and didn't have a central line dripping my poison into me. :::::We'll see what Celeste has to say about a feeding tube next time you see her.:::::

I put on my happy face and took the hit. Four hours later I was out of the room and heading home.

Last night, I received an extra special gift from my chemo. My gift was a 103.5 fever. At about five in the evening I took a nap, during which I tossed and turned and felt as if I was getting a fever, but I didn't really know. Sometimes, I got the chills and sweats from the radiation and I figured maybe the chemo was getting to me a little, but when I woke up at eight, I was cooking. I called my doctor, who wasn't available after hours, and then I called the institute's doctor on duty. He wasn't very helpful, he told me I could take a couple of aspirin and see if my temperature went down or I could go to an emergency room. After a few aspirin and a couple of hours of my fever not going down, I went to the emergency room at Sacred Heart.

When they took my temperature it was 103 point something, and when they learned that I had chemo that morning they rushed me in. They also gave me an x-ray on my lungs and took my bloodwork.

I was scared. Susan and Stacy took me to the hospital and they looked scared as well. I knew they thought it was serious when they both went quiet, which is a rarity when they are together.

They ran me through the mill in the emergency room. In additional to the x-rays and the bloodwork they put me on an IV.

By midnight my fever had gone down and the doctor let me know that it was probably just a side effect of the chemo, since my lungs were clear and my bloodwork was good except for some abnormal readings of my liver.

By one o'clock in the morning, we were on our way home.

I slept until eight this morning and here I am, strapped in and ready to go.

The machine began its agitation. It didn't care how I felt. It didn't care anything about me. It did not care that I had a wife and three children as well as three grandchildren. It didn't give a damn. It just did what it was told to do and shot me over and over again, day after day.

It certainly couldn't commiserate with me about how I felt. It purely did what it was told by some logarithms set forth by somebody.

I kept thinking about the ornament Jenn had sent. Faith, Hope, Strength.

I needed all three of those now.

I have faith, I believe there is a higher power and I have faith that the power has a plan for me and for all of us. :::::What if the plan isn't what you want?:::::

I struggled with hope. :::::What makes you think you deserve to hope? Why you and not somebody else?:::::

Did I do the right things throughout my life that allowed me to hope? I don't know. I always struggled with my decisions and how they may have hurt others. :::::Does it matter if you did the right things?:::::

In my work in the Navy, I always did my best. I always took each person's wants, needs and desires into consideration and tried to help them the best I could within the rules, but in the end the needs of the service almost always took precedence.

As I got more and more senior, the less I saw of actual people and the more I relied upon the rules. By the time I was a Lieutenant Commander, I was almost required to make all decisions based on the facts and not upon emotion. :::::Made it simple for you didn't it. Not your problem, not your fault.:::::

By the time I was a Commander, I was making decisions that impacted a significant number of people whom I'd never seen or never would see. :::::You never met some of them and you made decisions which altered their lives. Your decisions sent people into danger every day.:::::

That was a problem for me. Even though I used the books and rules, I tried to temper those decisions with empathy for others. I tried to understand the motivation of others and be more lenient or give them a break. I always wondered if that was the right thing to do or should I have just blindly followed the rules.

The decisions I've made in the past make me wonder if I deserved to hope. :::::Why are you so special?:::::

How many young men and women walked into my office with the hope that I would be understanding and lenient with them and I was not? I could justify it by saying I followed the rules and by feeling that the decisions I made about others would be best for them and for others. :::::Were they really?.:::::

When I sent a person out to sea knowing that his father was ill and that he would probably never see him again was it the right thing to do? If I didn't do it, what about his shipmates? Was it fair to a person's shipmates to send them to sea short a person so they were taxed with the additional work? :::::There are no easy answers.:::::

What if everyone had a reason not to go? What if nobody wanted to go? I mean really, does anybody really want to go to sea for Christmas? Let's take a vote. Very few would go. It was my job to ensure we had enough people on our ships and that they were ready to go. :::::What if they had a war and nobody came? What if?:::::

It was about the big flick of the nation and not about the individual. But what was the cost of that to everyone? Sometimes I hated it. I hated looking into someone's eyes and letting them know that they were going to sea and would not see the birth of their child. I hated it, but I did it and I did it without hesitation. I believed that it was for the greater good. :::::And you could always justify it by saying you'd been through it yourself. Like that's a good reason.:::::

I made the decision to discharge hundreds of young men and women for administrative reasons, from illegal use of drugs, to personality disorders, to violating "Don't ask, Don't tell." I did it because it was required by the rules. Did I believe in it? I did. I believed it was needed for good order and discipline but I wondered how my decisions changed the lives of those young men and women. Did I do it too cavalierly? Did I made good decisions?

Did I deserve to hope? :::::Maybe.:::::

One decision particularly disturbed me.

It was a Friday afternoon at the Submarine Base in Pearl Harbor, Hawai'i. I was the Executive Officer of the Submarine Support Command and was responsible for making, with my Commanding Officer's permission, almost all personnel decisions for all the submarines assigned to Pearl Harbor. I received a call.

"XO, this is the XO of the New York City. I took MM1 Johnson to Non-judicial punishment today and the Captain kicked him off the ship and told him to report to you. Has he shown up yet?"

The XO's voice clearly let me know he was stressed. "I haven't seen him," I said.

"You better go find him. I'm worried about him."

"Why would I find him? He's not assigned to me. He's yours. You find him. I'm not taking him until he checks in here. He's assigned to you."

"The Captain said he wants you to find him."

"Screw that. He's yours. When I get him delivered to my door, he's mine."

"He sounded depressed when he ran off."

"Then you better go find him and you better do it quick."

I hung up and forgot about our conversation until Saturday night when I got a call that MM1 Johnson had killed himself.

It haunts me. Could I have saved him? Did I do everything I could have done? I could have had a hundred people out searching for him within ten minutes. Would I have found him? I don't know. Was he my responsibility? No. But was that good enough? No. I could have done more but I didn't because of what? :::::It was your ego. You could have done more. Maybe you could have saved him. You could have stepped in and tried even though he wasn't "technically yours." Isn't every human life everyone's responsibility?:::::

From that day forward I made decisions differently. I still made them, but I tried to use more compassion. I learned that doing the right thing by the book didn't absolve me from trying to do the right thing for the individual. But in the end a rule was a rule and I still made hard decisions that adversely impacted individuals for the greater good. :::::Hard ass.:::::

I was responsible for those decisions. Did I deserve to hope?

How about those that I had saved because of following the rules? How about the many I sent through rehab before I discharged them?

What about all the people I got help for whenever they said "I might do harm to myself and others."? I'm sure a vast number were playing me and the system, but I sent them to the psychiatrist because I didn't want any of them to hurt themselves or anybody else. Did it save any lives?

How about the many young men and women I stood up for to ensure that they received equal treatment? Did it save any lives?

How about the thousands of Sailors that I counselled over twenty-eight years. I helped them. Didn't I?

How many people did I track down to make sure they were okay? A lot. :::::But not all.:::::

Did I save more than I lost? A lot more? I always tried to live my life the right way. I never intentionally hurt anyone but I would pull the trigger when necessary. :::::And look where you are now.:::::

Did any of it mean anything? Why was I balancing everything out? Probably because I needed to feel that I deserved to hope.

Did I deserve anything other than to pass away? Did I deserve to hope that I would be in the two of three that would survive this? What about number three who would not survive, did he or she deserve it any less? Didn't he or she deserve to have hope? What made me any better or any worse? :::::Nothing, you aren't any better than anyone else.:::::

I wanted hope. If I had known that the things which didn't turn out well would have gone bad, I wouldn't have made those decisions. :::::That's true, you never intentionally hurt anyone.:::::

What about what I did to Susan? Did I deserve to hope at all?

Did I deserve to hope or does my life up to this point not deserve hope.

How did the scales balance? Did they? Did it matter?

Lord please help me.

I'll try to do better for you. Please let me survive.

Day 17 – Wednesday - June 22, 2011

My machine's best friend Mike was dressed in Navy blue and grey camouflage scrubs. "It's halfway today! How do you like my scrubs, I'm wearing them in honor of you."

"Jeez Mike, those are hilarious, you look ready to join up."

"Not this kid. I like it right here. How are you feeling?"

"Fine." He didn't even have to tell me to move around anymore. I hit my marks without even trying. "I'm almost half way home."

"I heard you went to the hospital the other day. Don't worry, that happens a lot."

"It scared me. I didn't know what was going on. I don't think anybody knows what was going on."

"Sometimes it just happens that way."

"That's a comfort," I said as he tightened the last bolt.

My dear blinking friend began its warm up sequence and I began to space out. Once upon a time it scared me but now it had worn me out.

I think this was called de-sensitivity training. If you saw pictures of disturbing images long enough you eventually became accustomed to the pictures and they didn't upset you as much as they would the first time you saw them. With enough time and repetition you could get used to almost anything.

That's what was happening to me now. Once upon a time I was deathly afraid of this machine. Now, although I didn't like it and I was still afraid of it, I just walked toward it every day. Day after day. My sensitivity to this damn machine was now almost gone. Now that I knew it wouldn't kill me on the spot, as I once feared, I just marched toward my fate as directed. My heart rate went up a little, but not much.

Yesterday I received a package from my mother. It's strange how many packages and gifts I get now. I'll admit that they give me comfort, but they also scare me further. It's like people around me have to do it fast because they might not get a chance in the future.

It was a scrapbook of pictures from my youth. :::::Oh boy, you know it's getting bad when they send you pictures of yourself as a kid to make you feel better.:::::

There I was in my Lederhosen, with my brother Bob and our German Shepard Fritz, for a Christmas picture. I hated Lederhosen. Did they itch! From the minute I pulled them on, I remember sweating profusely. They were grey colored deerskin with black trim. On the lapels of the coat were deer ornaments made of bone. My brother and I wore matching outfits. At the time of this picture I was seven and he was four. :::::Weren't you cute. You were husky even back then.:::::

Even though my brother and I lived in the same houses for the first thirteen years of his life, we really didn't know one another. I was the oldest and he, as the middle child, was always at odds with me.

When he was seven and I was ten, he decided that he wanted the upper bunk of our bunk bed. I refused and my parents backed me up, so in order to get what he wanted, he took out some of the slats on the bed. That night I climbed up and jumped into the upper bed whereupon the remaining slats broke in half. I along with the mattress landed on the lower bunk. Unfortunately for Bob, he was already lying down and I crushed him and gave him a nosebleed.

Of course, he screamed and my father came running in, and Bob got what he wanted. From then on, he slept in the top bunk and I slept on the bottom.

As we grew older we grew further and further apart. Since I was about three years older, we had a completely different set of friends in Wisconsin. My friends were all into sports and his friends, I think, were just into running around. He really had no interest in me and I had no interest in him. We were never in the same school together in Wisconsin that I can remember. When I was in middle school, he was in grade school and when I was in high school, he was in middle school.

When we moved to Belize we went to the same school for a while but while he was out goofing off after school, I was mixing cement and hauling wood for the hotel. We crossed paths on the way to school every morning, rode the same boat to and from school occasionally and ate dinner together sometimes but we never really talked. I was not interested in what he was interested in and we never got close even though we were pretty much the only gringo kids on the island.

I do remember him catching a sea turtle which was about two feet around. At some point, soon after he caught it, he, along with my father, decided that we needed to make a pen for it. Bob and I pulled down some branches from a nearby tree, cut them up and made the pen, in which he placed the turtle. A couple of hours later we found out that the sticks were from a "poison wood" tree, some strange relation to poison ivy, only much more vicious. I remember our faces and bodies being swollen and itching all over from the poison wood. I hated that stuff. :::::Kind of set the tone for your whole early relationship didn't it?:::::

He and I took different paths. He messed around with creatures. By the time I was fifteen I was chasing girls.

He was thirteen when I ran away and moved out semi-permanently from my parents. Occasionally we ran into each other and said hello, but I don't think we ever sat down and talked.

When I left Belize to join the Navy he was fifteen. I don't think I saw him again for maybe five or six years. By that time, my father had sold the hotel, they had all moved back to the United States and my brother had been put up at a military school for his senior year in high school. After military school he went to the University of Illinois and got a chemical engineering degree. My younger brother had become a smart guy.

After he graduated from college, he joined a chemical company. He has been working with them for about twenty-five years. He is Global Director there and continues to be a smart guy.

Over the past twenty-five years we have seen each other occasionally and have become closer over the phone. On top of being a smart guy he's also a good guy and has lived a completely different life than I. We couldn't be more different.

He is the guy that when he sees the sign that says "Do not go beyond this point!" believes that it is a direct invitation to go beyond that point. When it says, "Don't step here!" it means that is where he is stepping. When it says "Don't ski beyond this point!" he looks at it, thinks about it and goes beyond it. I am a rule follower, he is the rule breaker.

I am the guy who has been married for thirty some years, he is the guy who has never been married.

Over the years, when we have seen each other, I have seen a parade of very attractive women with Bob. They are all very nice, but somehow it doesn't seem to work out. When we lived in Hawai'i, he'd come out to see us almost every Christmas. Every year he brought a new girlfriend with him and like clockwork, two weeks after the trip, he would break up with them. It got to the point that I wanted to get t-shirts printed up, ones like touring rock groups have. They would say "Bob's Hawai'i Tour" on the front and then have a list of girlfriend names and years on the back for each and every girlfriend he brought to Hawai'i. The list was so long that I would have had to order extra-long t-shirts.

In the 1980's and 1990's he called those women "Arm Candy" but now I think he is getting a little lonely. Now when he is looking for a long term relationship I think it's a little harder for him. Once you do things your own way for thirty years, without the help of anyone, it is difficult to change the way you do things. For me marriage is an exercise in compromise. I don't think he really wants to compromise or defer to anyone yet.

Even though we are so different, we are now becoming good friends. Since he learned that I became sick he has been here to support me and I think we are truly becoming the brothers that we want to be. I appreciate him now more than ever.

It's never too late.

:::::Maybe. You don't know do you?:::::

Day 18 – Thursday - June 23, 2011

"Whoo Hoo. Go ahead Mike, screw me in. It's halfway day in my mind."

"I thought yesterday was halfway."

"To me it's today. I have less than halfway to go after today. It's all downhill from here. What no fancy pattern scrubs today? Just plain old green?"

"All my fancy ones are in the wash. Thought I'd be daring and not wear anything wild. That really messes with everyone's minds." He finished screwing me in.

"If you wore the Navy ones again, we'd have to talk about you enlisting."

"Sorry, I'm too old." Having finished, he turned and walked away.

Halfway night is always special for every Submariner I know. When you serve on Strategic Missile Submarines there are two crews, Blue and Gold, and you switch on and off approximately every three months, submerging for about ninety days at a time. When you are out punching holes in the ocean at an unspecified depth and at an unspecified speed for three months at a time you have to do things that keep you busy. Halfway night is one of those things.

Halfway night is a night when some of the rules can be broken onboard the ship. It is a night when you can bid for the Executive Officer or any other officer (with the exception of the Captain) to be your personal slave for a couple of hours. It is the night you can bid to put a pie in the face of somebody who annoys you, just because, without retribution.

It is the night when general good natured debauchery takes hold. Can you imagine *Mardi Gras* within the closed spaces of a submarine? Sometime during halfway night it also involves gambling, beauty contests in drag and possibly alcohol. That was halfway night.

To add a little spice to the night, I usually started out by messing with the ship's Executive Officer during the day.

It is a time honored tradition of all Yeoman worth their salt to steal the Executive Officer's door and hide it on halfway day. The Executive Officer should know it is coming, it happened every patrol, and you would think they would be aware, but it is easy to get them out of their stateroom with some high level help.

"Captain, can you take the XO for a walk back aft? I need to steal his door," was all I had to say to the Captain.

"Sure, in about half an hour I'll take him back aft for about forty-five minutes. Make sure you hide it well."

"Thanks Sir."

A few minutes later the Captain walked by the door of the Yeoman's Shack, about twenty feet away from the XO's Stateroom, with the XO in tow.

As soon as the Captain and XO walked by, I got up from my chair, screwdriver in hand, and headed for the XO's door. It had about twenty screws and took about ten minutes to get it off. That was the easy part. The real question is where you were going to hide it. You would think that it wouldn't be hard to find a missing door on a submarine, but if the crew tries hard enough, you will never find it. Everyone has their own special hiding spot.

Once I got the door off, I grabbed it, it weighted about seventy pounds, and hauled it back aft to the Missile Compartment to hand it off to a Missile Technician for hiding. There is lots of room in the missile house to give a door a new home. "Here you go, Gleason, take good care of it."

"You got it, Wendt."

"I'll let you know if I hear he's headed your way," I said.

"Please do, but it will probably be long gone and in someone else's hands."

And so it went. We would play tag with the door, passing it on from one of us to the next, hiding it for a short while and then passing it on again.

By the time it was passed on to the third person, I had no idea who had the door. When the XO returned from his trip back aft with the

Captain and discovered his door was missing, he immediately assumed I was the culprit.

"Wendt, do you have my door?"

I could honestly say, "No Sir"

"Do you know where it is?"

"No Sir, I do not."

"I know you stole it, Wendt. Go and get it for me. That's an order."

"Sir, I don't know where it is."

"Go and find it or you will pay."

"Sir, you can't make me pay for what I didn't do."

"Get out of here and go find it."

"Whatever you say," I replied, "but I don't know where it is."

"Find it."

"Yes Sir!"

"And another thing, how come when you say 'Yes Sir' it sounds exactly like you are saying, 'Fuck You'?"

"I don't know, SIR!"

"Get the fuck out of here and find my door!!!"

I went back to my office and sat down.

Thirty minutes later I left my office and started looking for the door but somehow I couldn't find it.

After an hour of walking around and not finding what I didn't want to find, I returned to the XO's Stateroom and low and behold he had two of the guys who worked for me standing at attention in front of his door blocking my way.

"XO, can we talk?" I asked

"Sorry, I can't hear you, my door is closed."

"You don't have a door. Somebody took it."

"These two guys are my door. Duffner, Williams, left and right face."

They did as told and left a passage for me to walk into the XO's office. As soon as I got in, he said "Duffner, Williams, right and left face." Thereby shutting the door behind me.

"How can I help you, Wendt?" He stared at me with a smirk on his face.

"I couldn't find the door. I don't know who has it."

"That's okay, I have a new door. These two have kindly volunteered to serve as my door. They will be here twenty-four hours a day until my door is found."

"Nice work, XO," I said, "but I don't know where your door is and it's not fair to my guys that you are assuming it's me who has stolen it."

"Who do you think you are dealing with, Wendt? I went to the Naval

Academy and you didn't even graduate from high school. I'm a Lieutenant Commander and you are a Petty Officer. I will always be smarter than you." He had a shit eating grin on his face.

"I didn't realize how smart you were, Sir. Why don't you take a walk for a half hour or so and maybe your door will return."

"Sounds like a good idea," he said. He stood up, ordered his makeshift door to open, and left, ever convinced of his superior intellect.

I made a couple of phone calls and had his door returned, good as new. I even screwed it back into place for him with the help of my two guys.

He came back an hour later and dismissed Williams and Duffner, seeing that his real door was now home. A few minutes later he called me into his office and shut the door behind me.

"Wendt, who do you think you are? I've been doing this a long time. Don't think you can pull anything over me."

"Oh, Yes Sir. Thanks for teaching me such a valuable lesson."

"Stop saying 'Yes Sir' so it sounds exactly like 'Fuck You'."

"Yes Sir! Am I dismissed?"

"Get out of here before I get pissed."

"Yes Sir," I said, once again with a little extra on the "Sir," and exited his stateroom. I could hear him mumbling about how smart he was and how dumb I was as I walked away.

On the submarines which I served the XO's stateroom was connected to the Captain's stateroom by a shared head. The doors of the XO's and CO's staterooms faced each other and both opened inward. About an hour after the XO let me know how smart he was, the Captain came to my door.

"Wendt, how are you doing?"

"I'm fine, Sir."

"Looks like the XO got the best of you on that one."

"Yes Sir, but I'm not done yet. When you leave your stateroom would it be okay if I tied your door to the XO's door and trapped him inside his stateroom?"

The Captain chuckled. "Sure, he normally takes a nap around 1600 or 1700, is that a good time?"

"Yes Sir, thank you."

"No problem, just don't be too hard on him."

"Never, Sir."

Around 1600 the Captain came by my office. "The XO is napping and his door is closed. I don't need to get back in my office for a few hours. How about around 1700 I go up to Control and have them page the XO to report to me immediately in the Control Room."

"That would be great. Thanks, Captain." I stood up and grabbed some rope which I had prepared and headed to the XO's stateroom. His door was closed, as was the Captain's. Once I got there, I proceeded to tie the doors tightly together. Neither door could open from the inside now and there was no escape for the XO. He wanted his door back, he got it. I headed back to my office.

A few minutes later I heard the words over the general announcing system, "XO to Control."

About five minutes after the first announcement I heard the words "XO to Control, NOW," over the announcing system.

I left my office and headed into the passageway towards the XO's door.

I heard him screaming inside his stateroom "Open the fucking door." I ignored it. A saw the knob moving but the rope held the door securely in place.

Within a few seconds of my arrival, he picked up the phone and dialed Control. "Control, this is the XO," I heard him say. "Control, this is the XO, why is nobody talking to me?" "Open my fucking door."

After about ten minutes of noiselessly laughing my ass off and hearing him rant and rave, I decided to have pity on him. I knocked on his door. "XO, are you okay?"

"I am not fucking okay. Open the door."

"Sir, it looks like your door has been tied to the Captain's, I can't open either one. This could take a while."

"Just open it."

"Hold on, I'm going to need to get a knife," I said.

"Just fucking hurry, the Captain needs me."

"Yes Sir." I turned around and saw the Captain with a smile on his face.

"Set him free," he mouthed without making a sound.

I went to my office, got a knife, returned to the XO's Stateroom and cut the rope, thereby setting the XO free. When I opened the door, he was sitting at his desk, his face a dark shade of red. He seemed to be a little upset. Perhaps it was the realization that he was not always the smartest guy in the room despite his having gone to the Naval Academy.

"XO, are you okay? Who would do that to you?"

"You know exactly who. You made your point Wendt. Truce?"

"I don't know what you are talking about, Sir. We don't need a truce."

"Truce?"

"If you want one, Sir."

That night, during the halfway night festivities, I stole his skinny little mattress and pillows and stuck them in the shower and then took them to the freezer. Within an hour they were frozen bricks. At around midnight I took the mattress and pillows to his stateroom and made his bed for him.

By the time he got to lie down, about two in the morning, the pillows and mattress were nice and slushy.

I heard him scream but he didn't head in my direction. I guess he had enough for the day.

We both knew our places after that. I worked for him, but he understood that he should be nice to me or there would be consequences even if he was highly intelligent.

That was the submarine way. You never wanted to assume you were smarter than anybody else or there would be hell to pay no matter who you were. We are all in this together, no matter who we are. Nobody is alone in all this. None of us is too big to take the fall. :::::Tell me about it.:::::

I snapped to. It was nice to get away for just a while and not think about what was going on inside me. I have an appointment with the nutritionist and Dr. Baker in a couple of minutes and I know that Celeste is going to have a piece of me. So what that I'd lost more than she wanted me to?

:::::So what? How about a tube?:::::

Not going down.

A couple of minutes later I was unbolted and went to see my favorite nutritionist in the whole wide world.

Day 19 – Friday - June 24, 2011

"Well Steve, what do you have left? Sixteen more?" Mike asked, as he quickly tightened the bolts, making sure I was nice and snug.

"Yep, are you tired of seeing my face yet? Really? Mickey Mouse Scrubs?"

"Nah, it's nice to see your face every morning at the same time. You are always one of my first for the day. Sixteen isn't so bad considering where we started. As for Mickey, you know he lives in the happiest place on earth!"

"And here I thought the happiest place on earth was right here under my mask."

"I heard you had a couple of doctor's appointments yesterday. How did they go?"

"If you heard I had a couple of appointments then you probably know how they went. They went okay. Doctor Baker says I'm doing fine but Celeste ripped me for not eating enough."

"Man you gotta eat. Your mold is getting looser and looser. I can't have you moving around in this thing. These zoomies that we are shooting into you are very precise and I can't let you move. We don't want to miss any spots. We have to wipeout everything that could hurt you. I've seen them put tubes in people before. I recommend you try and find a way to get calories in."

"What, did you and Celeste have a little discussion before I came in this morning? I told her yesterday that I'd try to eat better. I drank four of those protein drinks since my last appointment and I'm going to get more down."

"Got to keep your energy up. We are a little more than half way but we aren't done yet. I'm rooting for you. Everyone is."

"I know."

"Then eat or drink or whatever. I'm sure it hurts when you swallow or put something down your throat, but do it for the sake of yourself. I've been doing this for about ten years and I can tell you that eating makes a difference, just like attitude makes a difference."

"Got it. You might have a future in this line of work."

"Maybe." He finished screwing me in and walked away without any further conversation.

The machine started moving. Today it appeared to me to be some sort of magic wheel, the ones you see at a casino with numbers 1-100. You put your dollar down on the number you wanted and the pretty girl dressed in a skimpy outfit, with her double D's sticking out, spun the wheel. Round and round it went, where it stopped nobody knew. It started clicking quickly at first and then eventually the clicking slowed down - tick, tick, tick.

I'm still here, fighting the fight. :::::But you have to fight harder. You're almost there. Gotta listen up to everyone. They are experts.:::::

How far am I from where I started?

My operations are over. :::::No more of that for now.:::::

My throat and neck hurt all the time. I started putting aloe on my neck as Dr. Baker suggested, but the radiation is literally burning the skin on my neck. The wattle which I started to get a few weeks ago is getting larger. It's like I have a goiter down there. :::::Boo hoo.:::::

Inside my mouth is no better. My throat hurts, period. It is sore enough that I'm done eating anything real. I was down to a couple of drinks per day. :::::Got to put in seven or eight a day.:::::

The good news about the protein drinks is that their taste is muted, the bad news is that they make me want to throw up. The radiation has killed most, if not all, of my taste buds.

I've lost twenty some pounds, more than twenty-five, at this point. Yesterday I told Celeste that she looked like she could eat a little more as well and that when she gained some weight, I'd work on gaining some weight. She did not look amused. :::::Good idea, give the people that are trying to help you a hard time.:::::

Dr. Baker isn't totally committing one way or another at this point. His words are not quite as optimistic as they were when we met for the first time. Yesterday he said, "You are doing well and it looks promising." I don't blame him for not committing, I think he knows that we are just playing *Spin the Wheel* here and he's the large breasted woman in charge of spinning it. He knows that two out of three with this cancer will make it and one will not. I'm convinced that he doesn't know who the one of three is, even though he's been doing this for thirty years and is obviously brilliant.

You can call it whatever you want. *Spin the Wheel*, a *Crapshoot, Russian Roulette*. :::::Two out of the six chambers have a bullet. Go ahead, spin the mechanism and pull the trigger.:::::

It doesn't really matter. Those are just words I use to try to comprehend what is going on and to let myself know that I need to hope. :::::Of course you have hope. If two of the six are loaded, that means four of six are not.:::::

Mentally is where this is most taxing, both on myself and on my family.

I'm the kind of guy that doesn't want to get overly enthusiastic. I don't want to get too high. I'm always afraid that if I get too high something or someone is going to come along and take my knees out from under me and bring me down. :::::That's stupid.:::::

I don't feel as if I deserve to be too high and I definitely don't want to go too low, so I do my best to maintain a level keel but honestly right now I'm feeling as low as I have for a long time.

I don't know if it is my mental state dragging my physical state down or if it is my physical state dragging my mental state down but I know they are both being dragged down. :::::That is some stinking thinking Steve. Get over it.:::::

I'm not quitting though. They can only zap me fifteen more times after today. That's it. Fifteen more times is my lifetime dose. I have had two chemo treatments and only have one left. No more after that. :::::That's better.:::::

I'm here now. I'm down, but I am not out. I've taken a couple of standing eight counts but nobody has counted me out yet and as long as I can move I am going to keep trying. I have a lot to live for. My wife, my kids, my grandkids, my son-in-law, my daughter-in-law to be, my friends.

Stephen, our son, who lives in Hawai'i called me yesterday. He is starting to call me every couple of days now. :::::Sound familiar?:::::: He and his girlfriend, Tracy and their child, Isaac, my youngest grandson are doing well.

He said he wanted to visit, maybe next week. I told him, "No, not yet, come and visit when I'm over this stuff and doing well." :::::That could be a while.::::

He said "Okay," but that he was going to call me every couple of days.

"Please do. I love you. Give Tracy and Isaac a hug for me," I said.

"We love you too Dad, take care." With that he was off.

Screw it, I am going to keep fighting. Isn't that what life is about? What choice do I have? I'm not going to give up, got to keep plowing ahead no matter how bad you feel.

:::::Atta boy, now you are talking. You have a lot to live for.:::::

Day 20 - Monday - June 27, 2011

"Just strap me in and let me go to sleep."

"You got it," Mike said.

:::::Jeez, it's Monday and you slept all weekend. Enough already.:::::

"Shut up"

"What?" Mike looked surprised.

"Not you. I was just talking to myself."

"Okay" He quickly finished making things secure and got out of that room.

:::::Great going. You'll probably get a call from the authorities today.:::::

"I said 'Shut up'. Let it go for a day please."

Day 21 – Tuesday - June 28, 2011

Round and round she goes.

This morning Stacy got up to see me off to my treatment. She gave me a hug and wished me luck. Even though she lives with us, she hasn't been spending a lot of time with me. I don't blame her. If I was twenty-one, I don't think I could deal with me either. Nobody wants to see a parent going through this. Whenever I see her she gives me a hug and asks how I am doing.

Stacy has always been our baby. She is nine years younger than her brother Steve and thirteen years younger than her sister Stephanie.

What's with all the S's in the family anyway? Steve, Susan, Stephanie, Stephen, Stacy, my son-in-law Sam, our grandson Stuart. We had a dog named Scruffy once. When I think about it now, it seems pretty weird but hey, every family has its thing. I wanted to name our oldest daughter Della after my grandmother but I didn't. Lucky for her. Stephanie broke the "S" spell with her youngest son Charles. I had a Father/Daughter counseling session about that, but what are you going to do? I told her she could have called him Sharles. She laughed at me. No go.

No matter how old Stacy is, she will always be my little girl. She was the only child that I was in the delivery room for. She came out sunny-side up with her face looking right at me, I was the first person she saw and I remember looking into her eyes as she exited.

When Stephanie was born Susan and I were only nineteen years old. We didn't have a clue. We also pretty much didn't have a dime. When parents don't have a clue they rely on what they know and both Susan and I were strict with Stephanie. By the time Stephen came along four years later we were semi-mellow, having been through it once before and having learned a bunch of lessons from Stephanie. We were also more well off. By the time Stacy came around, nine years after Stephen, she was essentially raised on auto-pilot and we were old hands who were much more financially stable.

We decided to have Stacy, I think, because Susan wasn't ready to be without children in the house by the time we were both forty. When Stacy was born, Stephen was in fourth grade and Stephanie was going into high school, but Susan and I were both only thirty-two.

At first I resisted the third child concept, but in the end I was along for the ride and did what Susan wanted. I couldn't have been happier. Just like Stephanie and Stephen, Stacy has always been a joy even though she and I are not afraid to disagree with one another.

Stacy thinks I am always mean. I guess I am.

When we moved to Hawai'i in 1994, Stacy was only three years old. We did not live on the Navy base, as we could have, but rather rented and later owned a house in Mililani, Hawai'i. I loved it in Hawai'i, Susan loved it in Hawai'i, Stephanie learned to love it in Hawai'i and married a man from Hawai'i and Stephen loved Hawai'i and is living with a girl from

Hawai'i, but Stacy has never really loved Hawai'i. She likes certain parts of it, but not all.

When we arrived in Hawai'i, Susan and I made the conscious decision that we would send our children to public Schools. Most of my contemporaries in the Navy sent their children to private schools. Some even sent their children to Puhnaho, where the current U.S. President went to high school. Puhnaho now costs upwards of twenty thousand dollars per year. As one of my bosses once told me - "I'm paying for my kid's college in high school." He was right, a ton of kids left Puhnaho with full ride scholarships at the next level.

Susan and I were both products of public schools and we had done okay. :::::Well, I was kind of a product of public schools.::::: Neither of us saw any problem with public schools.

I am pretty sure we made the right decision even though Stephanie initially struggled and eventually got a GED. It was, at first, hard for her acclimating from South Carolina. :::::Ya'all and all.::::: Stephen completely immersed himself without a problem. Stacy did okay but struggled at times.

Hawai'i is a different place and so is its school system. In Hawai'i almost anybody with means will send their child to private school and there are a significant number of those schools. Influential parents did not demand that the public schools be up to certain standards. Even most educators sent their children to private schools because they didn't believe in the very schools they taught in. When the educators don't believe, and they are the ones doing the teaching, where does that leave you? Also almost all politicians didn't send their children to public schools. When the people providing the funding for schools don't have a vested interest in all children doing well, that's also a problem. Senior military officers also, for the most part, didn't send their children to public schools because they felt they would be doing a disservice to their children and they expected and wanted better.

So who went to public schools when the children of teachers, politicians and the well-off didn't go to public schools? You can answer that yourself, but I can tell you that the people who taught and provided the money had no real interest in improving the system. In wasn't their kids on the line. In fact, they had a vested interest in not improving the system. The worse the public school system was, the better it was for their own children. The fewer highly educated youth in a small area like Hawai'i, the better it was for the private school kids who received the best education that money could buy.

I think one of the hardest parts for Stacy was that she was a very small minority in school. We lived in the Town of Mililani where most of the children were of any descent but Stacy's. In Hawai'i and in Mililani there was no majority. She must have felt out of place when she, as a blond haired, blue-eyed, tall girl, was the absolute minority. Ethnically speaking in Hawai'i there were Japanese, Chinese, Filipino, Korean, Polynesian, Hawaiian, Portuguese, Caucasian and a mixture of all of the above and then some.

I love the diversity of Hawai'i. When I look around in Oregon all I see is faces that pretty much all look the same, which was never the case in Hawai'i.

It must have been hard for my little girl. In every class picture she was the odd girl out. She was always the tallest girl and most times the tallest child in her class. She was also, almost always, the only kid with blond hair and blue eyes. I think it made her somewhat of a loner. Even when she got to high school, where there were more kids of her background, she didn't have a lot of friends. ::::::Maybe that's not it at all. Maybe she's just like you. After all, think of it, wasn't that your same circumstance?::::::

I will give Stacy this, she is a fighter. Probably learned it from her older brother and sister, maybe from her Mom and me. :::::She's like you in that way and you know it.::::: She does not fight physically but she never backed away from a verbal fight if she thought something was wrong. The other kid could be older, bigger and have more friends, but Stacy would not back down. She can cut just about anybody to shreds with her smart tongue and her whit. She will get to the heart of the matter and let you have it. No problem.

Even though she can rip you, she is also the most sensitive young woman I know and one of the most loving.

As she approached graduation from high school she decided that she was going to California to pursue her college dreams and dreams of becoming an actress. One of her friends from high school had moved to California and was going to school there as well.

This caused quite a ruckus with me. I did not want her to leave but she was committed and she had Susan's support.

We argued about it. When I look back I can't blame her for going. Susan and I were having a tough time at that point and she had been witness to all of our problems. I was gone at sixteen, why wouldn't she want to go at nineteen?

It dismayed me that she wanted to go all the way to California, away from all of her family, but I appreciate that she had the guts to do it.

She went, despite my dismay, and she did well and held her own. No acting, but she did work. Eventually she had it with California and moved to Oregon to live with Jan, Susan's friend.

Her moving to Oregon to live with Jan precipitated our move from Hawai'i to Oregon.

That move may have saved my life.

Thanks to Stacy, I am here getting treatment at an advanced treatment center and am fighting for my life.

"Okay, Steve, you are done."

"Done? Done, done or just done for the day?"

"You know better, just done for the day."

:::::Wishful thinking. How long did you think you were in there?:::::

Day 22 – Wednesday - June 29, 2011

The lights seem a little dimmer today inside my snug little cocoon. Perhaps it is me. I have less than three weeks of treatment left. :::::Well at least you called it a cocoon instead of a much more morbid name what starts with a "C" – coffin.:::::

Today was the last day of Michelle's treatment. When I met her she had a scowl on her face and she had one on her face today. :::::You can relate to that.:::::

Last Monday was Pam's last treatment. She went in and out without a word. Never said much other than hello and goodbye. :::::Can't blame her, don't want to get close to anyone.:::::

We never discussed Joan. I don't know if Michelle and Pam know what happened to her. I suspect they do. I don't want to know. :::::Chicken shit.::::: I know that she didn't come back.

That leaves me all alone. The four that were with me when this started are all gone now. :::::Not that you had a relationship with any of them.::::: They have been replaced by new people but I'm really not interested. :::::You should be. You are the one with a scowl on your face now. Maybe a kind word would help someone.:::::

Lying here, I feel as if the most important influence of my early life and the one who set me up for the rest of my life is here with me today, which is good because I need her as much as I have in a long time.

She has been gone now for almost forty years but I still hear my grandmother's voice in my head sometimes. It is there whenever I think about doing something wrong or something that I know she would never approve of. *"Stevie, you know that isn't right. You know that is wrong. You are better than that, Stevie. Don't do it!"*

:::::Man how many voices do you have in here?:::::

For my first thirteen years, my grandmother was the one I trusted the most. After my mom gave birth to me, way back in 1958, she didn't give me away or move away, even though having a child out of wedlock was a huge deal, not like it is today. Back then I'm sure it was a stigma to my mother.

After I was born I believe I lived with my grandparents until my mother married my father. It's not something I've discussed with my mother nor do I want to, we just keep it our little family secret that everybody knows and we all move along quietly avoiding the subject. I don't want to know and I don't want to hurt my mother by bringing it up so I just let it go.

As a child I was very attached to my Grandma Karas. She was one of thirteen children. She married my Grandfather Edward Karas during the Great Depression. He was one of twelve children. Both of the families were farming families in Wisconsin. In those days the more children you had, the more labor you had, plus the older children could watch the younger ones.

My grandmother lost her mother when she was young and the family was split up. She and a few of her sisters lived with an Aunt and Uncle until they were old enough to leave the Aunt and Uncle's farm. She did not like it at their farm. I think she always felt out of place and alone there. I also believe that she did her best to ensure that I did not feel the same way.

I don't really know when she met my grandfather but I know that they were married a long time, forty some years before she passed at sixty-five.

When my mother had me she was twenty-four. My grandmother had a special place in her heart for me and I had a special place in my heart for her as well.

Every year before she passed away, I would spend multiple weeks of the summer with her. I would help her in the half-acre garden she and my grandfather had. I picked vegetables and weeded. Once we picked the vegetables we ate some, canned some and froze some. Nothing went to waste. In the basement of their house they had a cellar which was full to the brim with canned foods including pears, peaches, cherries, pickles and sauerkraut, the aroma of which dominated the basement. She also had three big freezers down there where she kept frozen strawberries, blackberries, blueberries, beans, corn, rhubarb and peas. She had enough food for an army in that cellar. :::::She went through the depression and knew what it was like to be hungry.:::::

My grandmother was the best cook I ever knew. Her Thanksgiving spreads were unbelievable. :::::Don't you wish you could sit down and eat it all now?::::: The whole family would come together for her turkey with stuffing (inside the bird stuffing, not like most people do it today), ham, potatoes from her garden, yams from her garden, green bean casserole (beans from her garden), homemade bread and rolls, and silly green Jell-O with carrot shreds and miniature marshmallows which sounds so ridiculous today. For dessert she made traditional pumpkin pie with the pumpkins she raised and the best Red Velvet Cake I have ever had, even with the current resurgence of Red Velvet.

Just thinking about her food made me hungry in my brain. That's the only place I could really enjoy eating anymore. I didn't really salivate any longer, so I can't say that it made me drool, since that was gone. I can't say I could taste it, since that was pretty much gone as well, thanks to the radiation, and I really couldn't get all or any of it, perhaps the Jell-O without the carrots, into my stomach since my throat hurt so bad. :::::Yeah, but you can taste it in your brain right now can't you?:::::

It's ironic that so much of my memory of my grandmother involves food but actual food is pretty much unappetizing to me now. The stuff in my brain tastes better at this point.

My grandparents had six grandchildren, three from my uncle and the three of us from my mother. I was always my grandmother's favorite and I think it was because she and my grandfather pretty much raised me until my mother married my father.

Her soft spot for me created a lot of animosity within the family. Every summer I was the only grandchild invited over to stay with her and my grandfather before school started. During that time she would take me out shopping for new clothes which she did not do for any of her other grandchildren. :::::Maybe that's why your cousins don't correspond with you. You don't even know where they are!:::::

For Christmas I would get a couple of presents from my grandparents and all the rest of the grandchildren would only get one. For my birthday it was the same. :::::Maybe that's why!!:::::

At the time I didn't understand, nor did my brother or sister or cousins, since my out of wedlock birth was the dirty little family secret which we children were not allowed to know.

My grandmother and grandfather were also very Roman Catholic. Every Friday during the summer they would pick me, and only me, up and take me to a fish-fry since they only ate fish on Fridays, a tradition that seems to have gone the way of the dinosaurs.

I looked up to my grandmother in every way and listened to everything she said. I did so unquestioningly.

Whatever she told me to do, I did. She always told me to be good, mind the Ten Commandments and to always do the right thing. She said if I did, I would have a place in heaven.

I've tried Grandma.

My grandmother died unexpectedly on January 4, 1972. She went in to have a biopsy on her neck and somehow the doctor nicked her throat and she bled into her lungs uncontrollably. The night of the biopsy she suffocated to death in her own blood.

When she died, it was a shock to me. I had lost my best friend, the person who guided me most up to that point in my life, and the one I unquestionably listened to. I was just a kid then.

She, more than anybody else, taught me the first lessons that I would use forever. She molded me as much as anybody ever has. She taught me the lessons that I hope I pass on to my children and my grandchildren and I hope that they will pass them down as well.

To this day, I go to her for advice when I have a hard question.

I know intellectually that she isn't with me and that she can't answer my questions but I still ask. When I do, I get the response I know she would give me. It is a response that tells me to do the right thing.

Sometimes when I am getting ready to do something that is not right, her voice steps in, stops me in my tracks and makes me reconsider what I am doing. At the very least, it makes me ask the question: "What would my grandmother say if she could see me doing this?"

Today, I feel like she is right here, over my left shoulder looking at me and helping me through this.

Thank you Lord for loaning her to me. I need her as much as ever.

The machine stopped. Time's up. Only a few more to go.

:::::Oh shucks, you were just starting to love it.:::::

Day 23 - Thursday - June 30, 2011

Once more once. I am getting so tired of this merry go round. :::::Come on, Steve, it's the last day in June, the only full month of treatments. You'll be done by the middle of next month.:::::

Only twelve treatment days to go and then I am done with this. Or am I? What if it doesn't work? After talking to Doctor Baker today, he again said I am doing fine and they are doing everything they can at this point. The lifetime dose of radiation I'm getting makes this an all or nothing proposition. Either it works or it doesn't. If the cancer comes back all they can do is cut off some more of my tongue. I'm not good with that. I so much don't want that. :::::Stop the pessimism.:::::

Right now it feels as if they have taken out my throat. Everything seems swollen and when I open my mouth and look into a mirror I see how red and damaged it looks. In addition, since the surgeries on my tongue it is now lopsided. It's about an inch higher on the left side of my tongue than on the right. Looks strange, but it will do. My voice has stayed the same, but I'm not talking much anymore, it hurts a little when I do. :::::Everything still works, they might have damaged things, but everything is still working.:::::

I saw the nutritionist and I am now down another pound, but only a pound. I've been getting those drinks into me for the last week even though sometimes I end up throwing them up. Celeste was a little more encouraging and said, "Obviously you are making an effort." :::::A ringing endorsement.:::::

Swallowing is getting harder and harder. It's like swallowing in a desert, not much, if anything, to swallow.

At this point, when I'm sleeping, I wake-up every hour or so just to get some water in my mouth. My salivary glands are just about shot and the doctor said that it just may be that way from now on, but that everybody is different.

:::::Jeez Steve, you'd be bitching if they hung you with a new rope. What you have seriously beats the alternative.:::::

Day 24 – Friday - July 1, 2011

I looked around in the waiting room today, said "Hi" to everyone, introduced myself and smiled. I think I shocked them, a couple of their jaws fell open. I hadn't been overly communicative in the past. We didn't get to the nitty-gritty of who's got what and how long the treatments were before I got called in.

:::::Maybe next week. You've got three days off before you are back after today. No radiation on the 4th of July, just fireworks.:::::

Every day I keep pushing that boulder up the hill and every day it comes back down at me again. :::::Keep pushing, dumb shit.:::::

"Hey, I saw you wearing an Hawaiian shirt today." So Mike noticed. "I like it. It must be summer."

"I decided, in homage to the Hawai'i type weather, of which we get a week or two every year apparently, that I would wear Aloha shirts as long as the weather stays good. Maybe if I wear the shirts the weather will cooperate. It is, after all, the 1st of July. Plus I wanted to match you and your colorful outfits. But hey, look at you! Your scrubs have fireworks exploding on them. I can't beat that."

"Gotta explode for the Fourth of July. Are you getting a chance to get out any?"

"No, I don't go anywhere. I don't want to be exposed to people. I think my immune system is messed up. Plus I'm too tired. When it's nice, like today, I try to spend some time out on the lanai and get some sun."

"The lanai?" Mike was chatty today.

"Yeah. Sorry. The deck for all you Oregonians."

"Do you miss Hawai'i?"

"Oh Yeah, I miss it. I miss everything about it. I miss the weather. I miss the people. I miss my kids and my grandchildren."

"So why did you move here?"

"Cause I couldn't stand all the good weather, day after day after day after day. It sucks that every day is the same, 85 and sunny."

"You are kidding right?"

"Yes I am. I'm here because we all work for somebody."

"Ain't that the truth," Mr. Fireworks said. "Okay dude, you are all strapped in and ready to go. I'll see you in fifteen minutes."

"Aloha, see you in a few."

The machine fired up. It was all background noise at this point after four weeks and change. It was starting to remind me of the sounds of a submarine. You get so used to some noises on a submarine that you don't know how much noise is going on around you until the sounds are not there. That's when it becomes scary on a submarine, when the sounds change or stop. That's when you know something is going wrong. The sounds of this machine were the same as they ever were.

I stared up at the lights for a while before I closed my eyes and pulled the lever on my time machine.

Jeez, did I miss Hawai'i.

I miss the Sunday afternoon barbecue's we had when the whole family came over and everyone would sit down to steak and salmon.

I missed all the food. I missed the *Poke*, Ahi was the best. I'd stop by the local stores and get some *Poke* once or twice per week and bring it home and savor it after a run. It was always best along with a *Heineken* on my lanai in Mililani.

I missed the *Musubis*. They were rice with Spam on top, wrapped in seaweed. You could buy them at the local gas-station or 7-Eleven and eat them for breakfast. Oh yes, Spam, the national meat of Hawai'i. Somehow Spam tasted different in Hawai'i. They put it in everything. Spam and eggs for breakfast. Spam sandwiches. Spam fried rice was my favorite. I would get it at the Mililani Drive-Inn and bring it home to eat. So ono. Even McDonald's served Spam with rice for breakfast.

I missed the local fast food joints. Loco Moco and Zippy's. I loved the *Grilled Mahi with Garlic Butter* and the *Korean Fried Chicken*, *Kalbi Ribs* and *Chicken Katsu*. When you got them from the drive-in's or fast food joints, they all came in Styrofoam boxes and were called plate lunches. Each one came with two scoops of white rice and a scoop of *Hawaiian Mac Salad.*

You could get none of that here. They had pseudo-Hawaiian restaurants here, but none of them could hold a candle to the real thing. My test for any Hawaiian food place here was to see if the mac salad tasked like mac salad in Hawai'i but none of them could do it. I don't know why, they just did not, and if the mac salad didn't taste the same, then I knew everything they served wouldn't be right.

:::::Why are you doing this to yourself?:::::

In Hawai'i, you had the best of all the ethnic foods. The Chinese food seemed more real. Here you couldn't even get an order of *Egg Foo Young.* There were no real Korean places here, there were no good Ramen places. There definitely were no places where I could get *Lau Lau* or *Lomi Lomi Salmon.* I won't even talk about Filipino foods like *Lumpia.* They are non-existent in this town.

In Hawai'i they took the best of all foods and mixed them together using the influences of multiple cultures. Within a mile of where I lived there I could get any type of food that I wanted and it was good. Not so here.

This was the silly ass local brew, vegetarian, granola and gluten free capitol of the world.

:::::Why the hell are you thinking about food you idiot? You can't even taste food now. You definitely can't swallow any. You are thinking about all this and you want to feel like your mouth is salivating but it isn't. You are dry as a bone.:::::

I tried to swallow but I couldn't. :::::.Just relax Steve. Relax and swallow.:::::

I can't. :::::Close your eyes, concentrate and get your heart rate down. Relax.:::::

I can't. :::::Yes, you can!:::::

I need to get out of this fucking trap and sit up. Then I can swallow. :::::You can't get out of the trap. Relax so you can swallow.:::::

I can scream for help. I'm starting to choke. :::::Slow down. You are not choking. There is nothing to choke on. Don't panic. You are okay. Just relax. You can get through this. Your mind controls your body. The panic is self-created. Calm down. That's it. Relax. Take deep breaths, through your nose so your mouth doesn't dry up any more. Relax. You can do this.:::::

I can do this. :::::Yes, you can.:::::

I can do this. Inhale, Exhale. :::::That's it. Now try to swallow.:::::

I can't. :::::Yes, you can.:::::

I can. Let me try once more.

I swallowed! :::::Of course, you did. Stay relaxed.:::::

A voice came over the intercom, which I didn't even know existed. First time I heard it in four weeks and change. "Steve, are you okay, you seem to be trying to move and your breathing seems quick."

I cleared my throat. "I'm fine. Just taking a trip back to Hawai'i. I'm going for a run." :::::That's right, you have them fooled. Keep hanging in there. Only a few minutes left.:::::

Okay shithead, that's enough of that. You can swallow if you want. You just can't panic and try to make everything work. Relax. Relax.

I decided to sit on my lanai at my old house. I sat back in my lounger, kicked my feet up and looked around. I had a big yard, by Hawai'i standards. To my left I had about twenty banana plants from which I harvested bunches of apple bananas on a regular basis. A large plant had a bunch of about fifty bananas. After the plant produced a bunch, I cut them down and new ones would automatically spring up.

In front of me were Jabon, Meyer Lemon and Grapefruit trees. They were so prolific that I would give away hundreds of fruit per year to neighbors and those I worked with. Along the hundred foot back wall I had planted yellow Hibiscus which were all mature now and about six foot high.

Next to me was my dog Kona, a Sheltie. He wasn't very smart but he was the best dog I've ever had. Loyal to the core. Follows me everywhere I go now. Never complains. Gets up and greets me every day when I get home. Seems to like the crappy weather here more than I do.

:::::Now this is more like it. Just keep relaxing.:::::

On to Waimea Bay, my favorite beach, I went. I could feel my feet in the sand and the waves coming in and covering my ankles. On most days it was the most tranquil beach I'd ever been on, but in the winter when the big storms came in, it became a big wave surfing beach, one of the most famous in the world. I loved it there.

I would always go there early, 8:00 or 9:00 AM, in my old 1988 Jeep Wrangler with a bikini top and a broken gas gauge. I had to reset the mileage tracker every time I filled up so I knew when to fill up next. Since I always arrived early I would get a parking spot in the small lot. The best part about it was that when you got a parking spot on a Hawai'i beach you were golden. The beaches were always big enough that they could hold many times more people than the parking lots had spaces for, always guaranteeing you your own little world on the beach if you were there early enough to get a parking spot. This was true for every beach in Hawai'i that I knew of, except for Waikiki which was always overrun with people after eleven in the morning. That's why very few locals ever went to Waikiki. That was Touristville.

I sat there on my beach chair next to my boogie board and enjoyed the sand between my toes and the sun hitting my face.

:::::Now you are talking Steve.:::::

"Okay Steve, that's it for today," Mike said.

I slowly opened my eyes, not wanting to get up. "Just let me lie here for a while. Can't you give me a little more radiation today and just get this over with."

"Sorry, no. That's against doctor's orders. But I will let you come back Tuesday. Are you sure you are okay today."

"I'm fine. Just taking a trip while you guys did your thing to me."

Mike finished unleashing me and I sat up, stood up and walked away from my personal transporter.

"Aloha"

Day 25 – Tuesday - July 5, 2011

"Did you have a good long weekend?" Mike queried me in his usual upbeat mood.

"You know, SSDD."

"Say what?"

"Same Shit Different Day. We are going groundhog here."

"How much longer you got?"

"After tomorrow I am a one digit midget."

"Did you go with an Aloha shirt today?"

"Oh yeah, today I went Full Dress Aloha. Bright blue shirt with Birds of Paradise and other stuff. Made me feel a little better."

"Now you are talking dude, let me finish this up. How was your 4th? Did you see the fireworks?"

"No, your scrubs on Friday were the closest I got to fireworks. The fireworks aren't until after it gets dark, so I was long gone by the time they exploded. I think I heard a few of them when I got up to get a drink of water but no, not really. I'm too tired."

I could hear him tinkering with the bolts. "Okay we are done. See you in a few. Keep fighting."

He walked out of the room. No music today. A couple of seconds later my nemesis began to fire up.

"Stand-up and put out your hands," Emil Nunez the principal of St. Leo's High School in San Pedro said.

"You are not going to hit me with dat rope, Mon."

"Stand-up, I am going to lash you across your hands. You might be the biggest gringo in the school but I am going to lash you for your insubordination. Stand-up."

"I no was insubordinate and you are not going for lash me."

"Stand-up."

I stood. I was just over six feet. I towered over Principal Nunez, who stood about two inches over five feet. "I wasn't insubordinate. I just laugh when you say something. You are not going for hit me."

He moved toward me. "Put your hands out."

"Dat not going for happen. You not going for touch me." I looked around at the other school kids. We were all fourteen or fifteen years old, they were all smaller than me and they had their mouths open aghast. I didn't care. He was not going to touch me. "If you try for hit me with dat you are going to be sorry."

He moved in and started to swing his arm with the rope. I stepped forward quickly and pushed him and he fell onto the wood floor. I towered over him. "I done told you that you are not going for hit me. You can stay down der whiles I leave."

I left that school. Never went back again.

I didn't back down when my father called my girlfriend a black whore either. He grabbed that spear gun and I was gone. That was the last time I ever lived with my parents for more than a couple of weeks.

"Steve, we would like you to leave the classroom on Friday afternoons while we bring in some speakers from outside the school," Principal Ben of Wesley College in Belize City, my last chance school (really a high school), announced to the class.

"No, Mon. I stay right here. Dees are my classmates. I wan stay right here."

"These speakers don't want you here and neither do I."

"I no care. Why for I no can stay?"

"They don't feel comfortable talking to the other students while you are in the classroom."

"Why dat, because I de only gringo in dis classroom?"

"That's pretty much it."

"What dey going for say?"

"They just want to come in and talk about their beliefs for an hour every Friday afternoon."

"I be here."

"No, you need to go."

"We see."

That Friday, I was asked to leave the classroom for the last class of the week. I refused. The guest speakers wouldn't come in with me in the classroom.

"Steve, please go," the Principal said. "You are excused for the day."

"No, I stay right here." I looked around. I was now seventeen, stood six foot two and was in shape from mixing cement and lobster fishing. The other students with their epaulets, white shirts and khaki pants all looked at me with the same looks I got a St. Leo's. Those who would not teach with me in the room stood outside the door. I was somehow, no doubt, reinforcing their message.

"In my office." The Principal motioned me toward the door. A couple of other teachers were now there as well.

I stood and followed him out of the classroom. The guest speakers headed into the void. I really wanted to hear what they had to say.

I followed the Principal into his office.

"Sit down," he said, motioning me to the chair in front of his desk where he had taken a seat.

I sat.

"What are you doing? I told you that you needed to leave the classroom so those people could teach."

"Dat no right. Why I for leave? What can I no hear?"

"You don't need to be there."

"Dat my class and dos are my classmates. What da problem?"

"You can't be there."

"Or what?"

"If you insist on being in there, I will kick you out of the school."

"You no need for kick me out da school, I be gone."

I stood up, turned around and walked away. Never went back. They delivered my report card to me at the Bellevue Hotel, my exile home, a few days later. It read, "Steve is an above average student but this curriculum is not meeting his needs."

You aren't kidding, it wasn't meeting my needs.

Where did those school fights get me? They got me gone from two schools, that's where they got me. I was right but it didn't matter did it. :::::But I was right. Yes I was.:::::

Francis Linger, the owner of the Bellevue Hotel, sat me down in his office, situated on the Belize City waterfront. I worked at the Bellevue as a bartender for the last year or so while I was attending school. I kept working there for the past few weeks even after I left school. Francis was a good guy and he sort of looked out for me when he wasn't drinking or chasing skirts. Didn't seem to matter that I began to work there at sixteen and I was still not yet eighteen.

"Steve our till is coming up short for the last couple of weeks and Raoul tells me that you may have been taking money from it."

"No Mon, dat no right. I never takes no money from da till."

"Are you sure? That's what Raoul said when I approached him about money coming up short."

"It no me."

"Raoul said it wasn't him and he is the lead bartender."

"It no me and it only me and him, so he be lying to you. I never steal a cent from you. Once in a while I have a drink but you know that and I always asks you first. I no steal from you. Never."

"Okay, I'll be watching you guys."

"You no have for watch me. I no one thief. I never steal. Never. Even when I were broke and had nothing I never steal. I no do dat."

"I'll be watching you and Raoul."

I was pissed. I never stole from him and I never would. Him accusing me of that didn't work for me. "You no need for watch me, dis is my last week den."

"That's not what I wanted."

"Nobody is going for call me one liar. I done with you and dis place. Tanks for everything you do for me."

"You don't have to go."

"If you tink I could ever be da problem den I gots for go, Mon."

After that weekend I left and never went back. Raoul apparently kept stealing from him. Wasn't long before he was gone.

I hope Francis got what he wanted. Where did it get me?

:::::Where did that get you dumbshit? You were right and you were willing to fight for what you knew was right. That's where it got you.:::::

After leaving the Bellevue, I moved back to El Pescador, having burnt all my bridges at schools and at work in Belize City. It wasn't long before I joined the Navy.

The Navy was almost a perfect fit for me. My sense of right and wrong, for the most part, fit in right there. The three words they used: Honor, Courage and Commitment fit me to a tee. I didn't have to lie there. When I did my best and told the truth it always seemed to work out and I moved up rapidly.

:::::Yeah, you fought for what was right. Never afraid to have a fight if you thought something was wrong.:::::

"Man, what did you do?" I asked Petty Officer Shaw.

"I did what I thought was okay, Chief. It seemed right at the time."

"It seemed right at the time? Are you nuts? You entered a woman into the school reservation system as a man so you could get her the job that she wanted. You know that breaks about a thousand rules."

"I just made a mistake. I thought I entered her in as a woman, not a man."

"Bullshit. I have a computer printout here of all the times you tried to get her a medical job in the system. You tried over thirty times and then when it didn't work, you changed her to a male and booked it. Don't bullshit me."

"Sorry"

"Yeah, sorry. This is wrong. What are we going to do now? Do you have any suggestions? We are not going to do things the wrong way. I don't care if we make goal or not. We are going to do it right."

"I talked to the Chief Recruiter about it earlier in the day and he said it was okay and that what I did was right."

"The Chief Recruiter said it was okay? Who the fuck do you work for? Do you work for the Chief Recruiter?"

"No, I work for you."

"Do you think I care what the Chief Recruiter says? We are the job interviewers and we do this the right way. We don't lie, cheat, steal. We are always honest. I bet I say that at least once a week, probably once a day. Am I not getting through to you?"

"I thought it would be okay."

"It's not o-fucking-kay. If you ever do this again you are going to get busted. We do it the right way, understand?"

"Yes, Chief."

"I'll call you back in a few and let you know what I can do."

I hung up and called Naval Recruiting in Washington, DC. After I committed a couple of *mea culpa's* and begged for forgiveness, they overrode the system and gave me a medical job for the female. I called Petty Officer Shaw back and let him know.

Immediately thereafter I called the Chief Recruiter. I had enough of him.

"Master Chief Sutton, Chief Recruiter."

"Master Chief, Chief Wendt here. What the fuck are you telling my guys?"

"What the fuck are you talking about, Wendt?"

"You told Shaw it was okay to put a woman in the system as a guy?"

"Yeah. So?"

"Yeah. So? That's not the way we do it."

"It is if I say so, I am the Chief Recruiter."

"I don't give a fuck who you are. We are going to do it right. Stay out of my business. No more of your slimy recruiting deals, no more telling me to ask a kid if he ever used marijuana by asking, 'You never used Marijuana did you?' No more telling my job interviewers what they should do and how they should do it. If you have a problem with the way my job interviewers do their jobs, call me. Stay out of our fucking business."

"I'm the Chief Recruiter and I'll do whatever I want."

"Really? Let's go see the Captain."

"We don't need to, you just need to do what I say. I'm a Master Chief."

"Yeah, there is a need. We are going to do things the right way, not your fucking way. You stay out of my business."

That afternoon the Captain, the Master Chief and I had it out about who does what. The Captain sided with me and made it clear to the Master Chief that I and my people would handle the job interviewing and that he would stay out of it.

It pretty much made me a pariah to the regular recruiting guys. I didn't care. I was fighting for what was right.

"Lieutenant, you had better not go into the Admiral with that kind of attitude. That's a Captain you are having a problem with. Just pay him the money and everything will be okay," the Submarine Force Chief of Staff, a senior Captain, said.

"You know I can't do that, Sir. The book says that he has to ride submarines for two days a month in order for him to get full submarine pay. He didn't do it and I warned him that he needed to ride but he didn't find the time, so we can't pay him."

"Just fix it."

"I will fix it. I won't pay him. There is nothing I can do. I'm not going to fidget with the books. No way. That's not the way I work. You know that, and you can't order me to do it since it will be an illegal order."

"Lieutenant, I'm telling you that the Captain is going to go in the Admiral's Office and plead his case and the Admiral is going to tell you to pay it. You better get a new attitude."

"No thanks, I'm going to do what's right."

"Okay, you have an appointment with the Admiral at 1500. It's your ass!"

"I'll be there."

At 1500, I knocked on the Admiral's open door. "Request permission to enter."

"Lieutenant Wendt, come on in." I walked in. The Chief of Staff and the complaining Captain where already there.

"Steve, I've been discussing this sub pay issue with the Captain. What's up?"

"Sir, the Captain didn't meet his required submarine ride hours. He has to ride just like you. You know that you have to ride forty-eight hours per month and so does he. I warned him that he needed the ride time and that he would forfeit his submarine pay if he didn't, but he didn't ride. Now he would like me to pay him the money. Sir the instruction says that we can't pay him the money, it's cut and dried.

Admiral, you know that if you didn't ride I would have to take back the money from you and you know that each officer is responsible for his own ride time in accordance with the instruction. In my opinion we can't break the rules."

"You're right Lieutenant, don't pay the money. Thanks for upholding the rules."

"Yes, Sir."

"You can leave."

I stood up and headed toward the exit. "Close the door behind you please."

"Yes, Sir." I exited the door and closed it behind me. Somebody was going to get an ass-chewing and it wasn't me.

:::::So where did all that get you, always standing up and doing the right thing?:::::

It got me to a place that I could always sleep at night.

:::::Unless you got a bunch of phone calls.:::::

That's where it got me. Everybody knew where I was coming from and how I played the game. If you wanted to play loose and all over the place I was not your guy but if you wanted something done right, by the book, I was your guy.

:::::All you got was hated by a bunch of people.:::::

Not most of the people. Most of the people always did the right thing and they respected that I did the right thing.

I'd had so many fights in the Navy over doing the right thing. Just once I probably should have strayed from the rules but I couldn't do it.

How stupid was I?

"Steve how's it going in your new job as Windward Area Coordinator for the Youth Program?"

"It's okay, but I think I have a problem with one of the advocates who used to work here."

"What's that?" Jocelyn asked.

"I have this kid that we were looking after and one of the advocates was seeing him forty hours a week for almost a year before I got here."

"Really, forty hours a week? We are only supposed to see them ten to twenty hours a week max."

"Yep, this kid got over two thousand hours of services over the past year. I looked into it a little further, and the advocate who was doing it is now gone but he is dating another one of our advocates who is still with us and it turns out that the child receiving the services was his nephew."

"That doesn't seem right. Do you have the paperwork?"

"Yep, I made copies for you. If this is right, we charged the state more than sixty thousand dollars for this one child and we paid his uncle over thirty-five thousand dollars for taking care of him. This guy was getting paid to babysit his own nephew by the state. On top of that, I think under the state contract we can only service a youth for a maximum of one thousand hours. We need to give them back the money we overcharged them. We should probably give them back all the money. The uncle shouldn't get paid for watching his nephew."

"I'll look into it."

"Okay that's all I have this week. Same time next week?" I said.

"Yes, same time every week."

I let it go for a couple of weeks and we didn't discuss it. On the third week, I couldn't help myself.

"Jocelyn, did you look into the matter about the excess hours?"

"I did and it looks like something was strange but we can't do anything about it now. The person you took over for is gone, the person who did it is gone and the child is no longer being served. There is nothing we can do."

"You have to give the money back to the state."

"I don't think we can do that or that we have to do it."

"If you overcharged, you have to."

"I don't think so. It's fine."

A week later I found another job and gave them my two week notice. I didn't turn them into the state. I probably should have.

Where did it get me? I should have just shut up and kept doing the job.

:::::No way, you did the right thing. They did the wrong thing. They were the ones cheating. Take it easy on yourself.:::::

"Fred, I need to report something."

"Good morning Steve, what is it?"

"Look, I know I'm just a civilian now, but your XO, the job I used to have, is having an illegal affair with the Admiral's Yeoman and there is a good chance she is going to get hurt. I want to submit a formal complaint and have it looked into."

"Steve, you know that nobody is going to like this. Other people probably know about it and are just ignoring it. Just live and let live."

"No, I won't back down on this. Her boyfriend is a Marine with a temper and when he finds out and gets back from Iraq he is going to be pissed."

"Are you sure you want to report this?"

"You are the Inspector General for SUBPAC aren't you? I'm here reporting this. It isn't right and you need to do something about it."

"It's the Admiral's Yeoman. You are going to be messing with the Admiral."

"I don't care. I don't want anyone getting physically hurt."

After they ignored it for a while, I pressed ahead at the next level of the chain of command, the Commander, U.S. Pacific Fleet, and they eventually looked into it and the XO and the Admiral's Yeoman got fired.

I'm sure plenty of people were mad at me although they wouldn't dare say it since I had done the right thing.

I left that place a month or so after.

That was the last job I had before I got cancer a few months later.

:::::Where did all this fighting get you? What did all the trying to do the right thing do for you? You fought anybody at any time. Where did it get you?:::::

What I did was right.

:::::It didn't stop you from getting cancer did it?:::::

Is that the way it works?

Day 26 – Wednesday - July 6, 2011

Nine days and a wake-up. That's it. I hope I can make it.

:::::Steve, you are almost done. Just nine more.:::::

And then what?

:::::Then you go on with your life.:::::

What life?

:::::The one you have.:::::

Look what this has done to me.

:::::What?:::::

I look at myself and see one side of my neck is caved in and I got this lovely wattle under my chin. What the hell is that? It's not going away. I know it's not, no matter how much the doctor says it might.

:::::So what. You still have a tongue.:::::

Barely. It's crooked, one side is higher than the other.

:::::It still works, doesn't it?:::::

It does. What about my neck?

:::::What about it? You got what you got. Grow a beard.:::::

You know I can't, Susan doesn't want me to have a beard. She says that she doesn't like beards.

:::::Well then, I guess you have to live with the way it is. It's not so bad. Be confident.:::::

Yeah right. Confident. Look at me. People are going to look at me and see my neck and wonder, "What's wrong with him?"

:::::You can still be confident. You know how to do it. You did it for years. You used to go into a room and own it.:::::

That was a long time ago.

:::::Not that long ago. It's still in you.:::::

I don't know. I seem like a dinosaur now.

:::::So what, you are a little older but you still have a lot to give.:::::

Really? It doesn't seem that way. I am so worn out.

:::::Stop your incessant complaining. You are alive.:::::

For now. In nine days I get my last chemo. What's that going to do to me? You know what it did last time, it almost checked me into the hospital.

:::::That doesn't mean that's what's going to happen this time. That's what happened last time. You don't know what will happen this time.

You are going to make it through this.:::::

Do you know how I feel right now? I have never been lower physically. Never. I am so worn out. I struggle to swallow and it hurts when I do. My mouth is so fucking dry.

:::::Whaa fucking Whaa. Don't be a baby. You could be dead now. If they didn't do anything you would be well on your way to dead. You don't get to complain. So what, your tongue is weird, you neck is weird, your mouth is dry, you can't eat. And by the way, the protein drink thing and losing weight is on you. You know you can drink more of them if you want. So it hurts a little. Too bad. Too fucking bad. Take care of yourself, you can do it.:::::

What the hell happened to me? I can hardly taste anything anymore.

:::::Too bad. You don't need to taste anything to live. Anyways, you can smell things can't you? If you smell it then the flavor is almost there. Just the other day you were thinking about things your grandmother cooked and how you loved them. You thought about Hawai'i and the food. You were tasting food then weren't you?:::::

Kind of.

:::::Your memory of the food is just like tasting it. You can call up that memory anytime you want. Right now you can taste Sefarino Paz's bread from the bakery in San Pedro can't you? And you haven't smelled it or eaten it for over thirty-five years. But it is right there. It's in your mind.:::::

But…..

:::::But nothing. I don't want to hear it about your taste. You can bring up and taste anything you want. You have your eyesight, you have your hearing, well part of it, you can smell and you can feel.:::::

I can't feel everything, the left side of my neck is numb.

:::::I thought you said it hurt. How can it be numb and hurt at the same time? You can feel. Your hands work, they can feel. You get pain, that beats the alternative doesn't it?:::::

I guess.

:::::I guess? I guess? Let me tell you how lucky you are. You only have nine days more of this treatment and then you are done with it.:::::

Unless something goes wrong. What if it doesn't cure the cancer? They said that they couldn't do any more radiation or chemo. What if it isn't cured?

:::::You have got to look at this in a positive manner. No what ifs. No worrying.:::::

You know that's not the way I work. I am going to worry about it no matter what.

:::::I know you probably will, but that's up to you. You have control of you. It's up to you how you react.:::::

You are me. You know how I am going to react.

:::::How you react is up to you.:::::

You can't change fifty years of habits. I can't change how I am made up. I will always be worried. That's what I do. For all my life I worried about others. I know how to handle that, but this worrying about myself has overtaken me.

:::::Keep it calm Steve.:::::

I don't want to die. All I have done all my life is to try and do things for others, I don't deserve this.

:::::Nobody deserves it. Do you think your father deserved it? Your grandfather? Your grandmother? Your XO? Who deserves this shit? Nobody, but you got it and that's the way it is. What are you going to do? Give up?:::::

Sometimes I think it……

:::::Oh no you don't. You are not going to quit. You are going to keep fighting. No Sir. No quit. Who do you know who would want you to quit?:::::

Who do I know who would care if I quit? I could pass away right now and only a handful of people would care.

:::::That's not true.:::::

Who would even know or care? I'm an antique. I'm so old I probably can't even get a job around here. Nobody wants a washed up old guy anymore, especially one who has been sick. Who the hell would want me to work for them?

:::::First things first. There are plenty of people that want you. You can still contribute. Your brain is still intact. You are a smart guy. You don't need the money.:::::

Thank God for that.

:::::Yep, thank God for that. You are still important to a bunch of people.:::::

Really? Who would know or care if I went? I don't keep in touch with the people I worked with and they really don't care about me. I've burned bridges everywhere I went because I won't ignore things. I have to fight everyone.

:::::You would be missed all over the place. What about the thousands of sailors you helped throughout your career by fighting for them. You know anytime you see one they thank you for all that you have done for them.:::::

I haven't seen one forever.

:::::That doesn't change the fact that you helped them and they will miss you. What about all the young men you helped at the Youth Correctional Facility? You helped a bunch of them. You helped to get a bunch of them on the right path.:::::

Did I really?

:::::Oh yes you did. You gave your heart and soul to them and let them know that they were worthwhile. What would you say to them if they were talking like you are right now?:::::

I would tell them the same things you are telling me right now.

:::::That's right you would.:::::

But that's just talk.

:::::Oh no, it's not. It's real. And what about your family? They would miss you. They love you.:::::

I know, but they'd get over it. Look how I'm behaving now. I'm not as strong as I used to be. I don't want to be a burden to them.

:::::You'll be what you are. You won't be a burden. Your body works. You aren't paralyzed.:::::

But what if the cancer comes back?

:::::Then we deal with it. Steve you are tougher than this. You can't let this thing get over you like this. You have a fighting chance here. You are still living and still breathing. Ninety-nine percent of your body works the same. Your brain still works. Your heart is still beating. Your lungs are still breathing.:::::

Whatever.

:::::Not whatever. Your family loves you. You've had problems but you are still a good husband and father and grandfather.:::::

Not as good as I could have or should have been.

:::::That's the past. That's not now. What you do from now on is what you do from now on.:::::

I'm still so tired and worn out.

:::::I know, but you have it in you. Keep fighting this. You are a good man. You know you are.:::::

You think so?

:::::Here's what I think. You've always fought yourself. You always did your best even though you could have done better. Nobody is perfect. Nobody. You are too hard on yourself. You have lived a good life up until now. It's not time to quit that life yet. Susan loves you.:::::

I love her, but I need to be better to her.

:::::Then be better. Stop being so uptight. Relax. We are all along for the ride in this life and nobody gets out alive.:::::

Very funny.

:::::Not funny. Not even you, even though you have tried to do everything the right way. Nobody gets out of this alive and nobody knows when their time is up.:::::

What about what I did to her? How can I ever overcome that?

:::::You don't have to, she forgave you. She knows you didn't mean it.:::::

But still.

:::::But still nothing. Toughen up, you didn't mean to hurt her.:::::

I don't want it to end too soon. I still have things to do.

:::::Then do them because when it's done, it's done.:::::

I want more time.

:::::Nobody knows if you have any. I believe you are going to get through this though. Then what?:::::

Will I be better to Susan? Will I get to see my son get married? Will I get to see my grandkids more often and see them graduate from high school? Will I live to see a cure for diabetes? Will I get to walk Stacy down the aisle?

:::::Who the hell knows? I'm you, so I don't know. I know this – you are breathing right now. You are strapped into a machine but you are breathing and your heart is beating. If you're lucky you'll get the next breath and your heart will take another beat. There are no guarantees but everyone is trying to help you.:::::

I know.

:::::You have to do your part. You have to be positive and eat more. You have to know that you are worthy to keep going. Stop beating yourself over the head with a stick. You have done well. Be proud of all you accomplished in your life.:::::

Really?

:::::Yeah really. Really you shouldn't have made it this far. Think about it. Your mother could have terminated you. Your father didn't need to marry your mother. Sickness almost killed you a few times. A shark almost killed you. You served on submarines for years and any little mistake could have killed everyone. Think about how many opportunities you have for disaster in a regular life. Driving, living, just doing stuff. Any moment could be your last. And yet here you are.:::::

Yeah, here I am, bolted in while a crazy machine shoots some type of crazy radiation into me trying to kill me without killing me.

:::::That's right. That's where you are, but in about two minutes the machine is going to stop and somebody is going to come in and unbolt you and after that you'll have nine days left of treatment. That's it and then you never get to do this again. Maybe.:::::

Smartass.

:::::Up yours.:::::

You are right.

:::::I know BUTTERCUP.:::::

Day 27 – Thursday - July 7, 2011

"I saw you in the lobby. Nice shirt today!" Mike said. "Plus when I called you, you were actually taking to others in the waiting area. Nice job."

"I decided I could be a little friendlier. It won't hurt."

"Now you are talking. They all know you have been doing this a while and they need to know you are still standing. When are you going back to Hawai'i?"

"Who knows? Hopefully soon. Just got to make it through this first and then we'll see."

"You'll make it through this. Only eight days to go after this, right?"

"That's right. Thanks for keeping track."

"Somebody has to do it for you. What if we gave you an extra treatment? Don't want that."

"Don't worry, I'm counting."

"There are a lot of people counting. I spoke to Dr. Baker this morning and he says you're doing well. Celeste says your weight has been doing better. I see your wife is out there every day with you. I bet she is counting."

"She is."

"I bet she wants to get this over with almost as much as you do. Okay, let me get these bolts in. We padded your restraint a little bit so it fits tighter. Don't want you moving and the radiation hitting the wrong places."

"I appreciate it."

"Okay, we are all done hooking you up Steve, see you in a couple of shakes."

He left the room. Now it was just me and my mask and this machine. I once hated it, but I am starting to be grateful for it.

I have a lot to be grateful for.

They are going to get me on this machine eight more times and I'm going to get chemo once more but I'm going to make it through that. I am starting to see an end point for this treatment.

I know I'm going to hurt more before the next two weeks are over but I think I have enough in reserve to make it. I only lost a pound or two in the last week, I've been jamming in the protein drinks as best as I can. I looked at regular food yesterday, got a sniff of a hamburger, but that's not going to happen. Maybe in three weeks, maybe in a month.

As Dr. Baker told me, the damage from this radiation and chemo are cumulative, nothing is healing now. The bastards are still damaging me and shooting me up, doing their best to get rid of any possible remnants of cancer.

This morning I woke up mad at the cancer and not feeling as sorry for myself. I'm mad because it's trying to take away everything from me. It has been sitting inside me for years and then it made its move. Sneaky bastard.

I think it was waiting for me to be vulnerable enough to take me on. It was waiting for me to question myself and then it jumped on me.

Or maybe it was just waiting to get strong enough and then come out and kill me. Thirty some years it sat inside of me and then boom out it comes.

I can't figure it out. If it killed me, didn't it kill itself? I thought it was survival of the fittest. This wasn't survival of the fittest. This was kill the weaker and then in doing so, kill yourself.

Thank God I had people that were working to kill this thing inside of me off. It was trying to kill me and simultaneously kill itself but we were trying to kill it before it killed me so I could live. It was better to suffer the collateral damage and make it through then to not make it through.

There has been damage in this war. Major damage. Damage to me, damage to others around me. I would never be the same.

What doesn't kill you makes you stronger. I throw the bullshit flag on that silliness. Right now I didn't feel any stronger. Once I was in charge of hundreds of people. Once I was in charge of my body. Once I was in great shape. Once upon a time I was confident in my abilities and what I could do. I feared very few. I was strong.

That is gone now. This thing has humbled me. I am not in charge. I can do everything right, those around me can do everything right, but it can still kill me.

What doesn't kill you makes you humbler.

I need to be grateful and humble for what I have, for what I have been given to this point.

How many people have met the love of their life and have been able to spend over thirty years with them? How many people have had three wonderful children who love them and three terrific grandchildren?

How many people have been given the opportunity to go serve their country and go from a dishwater to a Commander? I could never have gotten there without the help of thousands of others.

How many people have been given the opportunity to go to college after having dropped out of high school?

How many people have been given the opportunity to help others?

How many people have been given multiple opportunities at life?

I have. I should be filled with gratitude for that.

Thank you lord for giving me all that you have given me. Thank you for my wife, my children, my grandchildren, the jobs I was given, the opportunity to serve others.

Please give me the opportunity to continue on this journey.

:::::Do your part.:::::

I'm trying.

:::::Try harder.:::::

"Okay, Steve, we are done for the day. Tomorrow is Friday. Let me get these bolts loosened."

"Woohoo," I said through the mesh. "Get me out of this thing. I have a wife to hug and a life to live."

:::::Now you are talking.:::::

Day 30 - Tuesday - July 12, 2011

The last four days were a blur. It's like I entered a state of permanent drunkenness. My head was spinning and all I wanted to do was sleep. I am officially getting my ass kicked. I was so out of it that I don't even remember going to the machine for two of those four days. But I kept moving ahead.

We are nearing the last of it. Only five more treatments after today. I am in the homestretch now.

:::::Pick your head up.:::::

I can't pick my head up, my head won't even move.

:::::Clever. Now you are thinking.:::::

Where am I going from here?

What do I want to do?

Should I just go travelling and see everything I want to see, knowing that I might not be around that long?

Should I just get in my car and go? Sometimes I feel like that's what I want to do. Can I just run away from all this when the treatments are over?

Can I just run away now? What if we went home and I got in a car and just drove off? What if I went south to the warm weather? Somewhere where I could just sit and let the sun hit me and warm me up all day long rather than this silly cold room with subdued lighting and an ice cold metal slab.

I've just about had enough of this.

:::::You've got to get through this. You can't leave. You don't want to leave everything behind.:::::

Why not? Why can't I just drive into oblivion? I would be less of a hassle. I could just drive to Mexico or somewhere deserted, rent a room and live until I die without doctors or nurses or whatever. This stuff is getting ridiculous. I've been getting wacked on for five months now.

:::::One week left.:::::

I know. I would never stop now. That's only in my dreams.

:::::That's not your real dreams. You know it.:::::

I know, my real dreams are to be better and to live a happy, better life. My real dreams are to live the way I should. To be better to those that I know and to be better to myself.

:::::Keep digging. Go deep.:::::

To live a life for now, once I get through this. To stop putting things off, saying tomorrow, tomorrow. I've planned my whole life and now what? You can plan for tomorrow your whole life and then die and never do the things you want.

I've been saving my whole life. I've been putting things off saying tomorrow and when that time arrived I never had time to do them and I'd defer again. Enough with the deferring. Hell, when I was in the Navy I gave back over a year of vacation. Time I could have spent doing what I wanted to do. Spending time with my wife and family, travelling, just sitting, playing golf, reading, doing whatever I wanted to do. But no, did I do that?

:::::You didn't. You were stupid.:::::

You know I was. I want that year back to do things with it.

:::::You can't have it. That's past.:::::

Yes it is. Can't I mourn for it?

:::::Haven't you been mourning enough? Isn't it time for action?:::::

You are right, let me get up right now. Oh no, I can't. Somebody has me bolted in. Maybe I could yell and tell them to let me out of this ridiculous device now.

:::::Ha, ha. You know that's not real.:::::

I know I have to finish what we started here so I can have a shot at a life. A depleted life, but a life none the less.

:::::Depleted? Really? Is eighty percent of what you were, living at one hundred percent better than being one hundred percent and living at fifty percent, always planning for tomorrow and never doing anything today depleted?:::::

No it's more.

:::::That's right it's more. Now get to it. Cut the pity party.:::::

In a week or so, maybe a month. Can't even move now.

Day 32 - Thursday - 14 July 2011

"Nice outfit. My Little Kitty?"

"Not 'My Little Kitty.' What's 'My Little Kitty,' a mix of *Hello Kitty* and *My Little Pony*?"

"They are the same, aren't they?"

"What's wrong with *Hello Kitty*?"

"Nothing, thanks for helping me smile."

"You got it. See you in the blink of an eye." Mike turned and started heading off.

"What did you say?"

Mike turned back, "I said, I'll see you in the blink of an eye."

"Got it."

"Anything else?"

"No," I said. Mike turned and walked out of the room.

His saying "blink of an eye" brought me back to earlier this morning. I was thumbing through my Bible and I locked onto James 4:14.

Whereas you know not what shall be on the morrow. For what is your life? It is even a vapour, that appeareth for a little time, and then vanisheth away.

All our lives are vapor aren't they? The earth has been around for six billion years, man has been around for maybe one hundred thousand. There have been about fourteen billion people born on earth. Fourteen billion Steve, and you are one. That's it, just one out of fourteen BILLION. One human in five thousand generations of humans.

:::::It's like you are a single grain of sand.:::::

I truly am a vapor aren't I? Aren't we all? But even a vapor has some substance, doesn't it? Even a vapor has particles that influence things around it. How many particles are in a vapor? Probably depends on the vapor. What kind of vapor do I want to be? How many particles are left behind when the vapor dissipates? How long before the vapor dissipates? Where do those particles go? How do those particles in a vapor change others?

A vapor can be seen, a vapor can be heard when it comes out of a boiling kettle, it can be felt when it burns you, it can be smelled. Maybe it only lasts the blink of an eye, but in that time it can alter things and people for a lifetime, can't it? It can leave a scar, it can make you get up to remove the pot, it can make it impossible to see clearly. It can make you smile like the vapor being given off by a flower or it can make you hold your nose like the vapor being given off by a skunk.

A vapor can disappear and do zilch or it can make a lasting impression. What's it going to be Steve?

Do you just want to dissipate into nothingness without positively impacting anything or anyone in the future, or do you want to leave something good behind?

If I am a vapor, most of my substance is almost gone.

:::::But it's not all gone is it?:::::

How long do I have left? A day, a month, six months, a year, two, five? At five years you become an official survivor. Ten years? Fifteen?

:::::Maybe if you are really lucky!:::::

Your life might just be a vapor and that vapor might almost be gone but it isn't gone yet. You are still here Steve. There is less and less time that the vapor will exist every day, every hour, every second. What are you going to do with it? Curl up and vanish or take what is left and leave some goodness behind?

:::::It's up to you.:::::

Yes it is.

It's just the blink of an eye.

But at least I have a blink. For billions upon billions before me the blink is over. Time to make the best of what's remaining.

Day 33 – Friday - July 15, 2011

"Two left after today?"

"Yep, that's it. I am done next Tuesday. You ready to get rid of me?"

"Nah, you are good company. You never stay too long, you don't dirty the place up, you don't say much and you always leave on time. How are you feeling?"

"I'm feeling pretty rejuvenated. I can make it through the next few days with my hands tied behind my back, hanging upside down."

"Who are you? Houdini? I dare you to get yourself out of this mask after I put it on you."

:::::Mike has no idea that you get out of this mask every day, while it's still on, and go wherever you want. This is your own personal portal to wherever. Your Looking Mask.:::::

"Yeah, that's not going to happen," I said. "Maybe Houdini could do it, but it's a necessary evil so I'll let it be. I've withstood it for thirty-two days now, I can handle it for a few more."

"Do you want the mold when we are done?"

"Do I want the mold?"

"Yep, some people want it. They want to take it home."

"Why, so they can hang it up on the wall like some primitive art?"

"As a memento," Mike said.

"Yeah, no. If I took it home I would want to burn it, not keep it."

"You can do that too. We'll just throw it in the trash."

"Let's stop talking about it. I still have a couple of treatments to go after today and I don't want to jinx anything. I just want to make it through this and my last chemo so I can be done and then I can worry about what we will do with that mask."

I lay down and he promptly pinned me in. I'd gotten over the mask, but I hated what it stood for. If, and when, we got done here, I never wanted to come back. I never wanted to see this machine again. I never wanted to smell this place or see the sickly waiting room or chairs or pay twelve dollars every time I walked in. Never. Never. NEVER.

The machine began to hum and spin.

:::::What are you going to do after this is over Steve?:::::

I don't want to talk about it. We are too close to being done here. This last week has been physically wrecking me. I just want to get through it. I still have one hundred hours to go before all the treatments are done.

:::::Then what?:::::

Let me get through it first. If I talk about something, it is going to go bad. Remember Joan, she was almost done and BOOM. I haven't seen her since.

:::::That's not going to happen.:::::

I don't want to chance it. I'll just have to delay my decisions for a couple of days.

:::::What about Stuart?:::::

Stuart, oh Stuart.

My daughter Stephanie called yesterday afternoon and apparently my oldest grandson, who is thirteen, had a little skirmish with the law.

"Dad, I need your help. I know you are going through all this stuff right now, but you are almost done. I need to send Stuart to live with you guys. I don't know what to do."

"What's wrong?"

"Stuart was out a few days ago with a couple of his friends and he got caught writing graffiti on the walls of a school. The police picked him and his friends up and they said it was going to cost thousands of dollars to fix."

"What?"

"That's not all, apparently he and his friends got into the school and destroyed some stuff in an audiovisual room. They charged him with destruction of property and breaking and entering, and now he is going to have to go to juvenile court. I don't want him to go to jail. I need your help with him. He's been acting up over the last couple of months, running around with the wrong kids and not listening. I talked to Mom about it, but we didn't want to bother you, but this can't wait any longer. I need your help, I don't want him to go astray."

"You talked to Mom?"

"Yeah, but we didn't want to bother you with all the stuff you have going on. I don't want to do this, but I don't know what else to do with him and I don't want him to go to jail. If he comes to live with you for a while I know that you guys can help me with him."

"He's not a bad kid."

"I know, Dad, but he needs some help. He doesn't want to listen to me or his father anymore, and his grades went down the end of last year."

"Let me think about it. I'm worn out. When would you send him?"

"In a couple of weeks. I need to get a lawyer and talk to him, but I want him to arrange for Stuart to come and live with you. I don't want him to leave Hawai'i but I don't want him to go to jail. You worked in the juvenile facility and you know how it is. Please."

What could I say? This was my daughter asking for my help with my grandson. I loved them both.

"Okay, send him."

"Are you doing okay Dad? Your treatments are almost over right?"

"Next Tuesday they will be done, hopefully."

"You'll be okay Dad, I know you will."

"I will. I love you."

"Thanks for this, Dad. Stuart will be good with you. I just don't know what else to do."

"I know. I love you Stephanie. Be good. Call me."

:::::Now you gotta make it through.:::::

Day 34 – Monday - July 18, 2011

"One more day after today?"

"That's right, just today and tomorrow and then we are done with this. I am playing ping-pong against a curb."

Mike looked at me, puzzled by my last remark, but I guess he decided to let it go. "Do you have any chemo left?"

"One more tomorrow, as soon as we are done here."

"Is that it, then?"

"I guess so. That's what they say, except for checkups."

"I liked your Aloha shirt today. Let's get you down and bolted in, so we can be done for today."

"You got it." Down I went.

"See you in fifteen."

"Hurry up."

All I have left after this is tomorrow. This is my thirty-fourth day of this medieval torture. I also got to see Celeste and Dr. Baker today, as if this torture isn't enough.

Celeste let me know that I was now down to about two hundred and ten pounds. About thirty-five pounds from where I started five months ago. She was not pleased, but she was not unhappy either. She emphasized to me that I needed to start eating and that my throat probably wouldn't feel any better during the next week or so. Plus since I was getting chemo tomorrow, I probably wouldn't feel like eating for a week.

"Well at least I didn't need a tube."

"I thought about seriously forcing you to get one."

"As if you could. Never gonna happen."

"You are a big tough talker. Start eating or you could still end up with one."

Dr. Baker was his usual upbeat self. He felt up my neck and congratulated me for getting through this part but let me know that now we would start finding out if it worked or not. He told me that we would see me in a month and that I would see him once a month for a year and then we would go to once every two months and then to quarterly.

"Is everything looking good so far?" I asked

"Everything is looking very good right now. No signs of anything. We are hoping we got it all."

"Is there anything I can't do?"

"No, after this is done, what you do will be up to you. Do what you can. You are probably going to feel down for quite a while but about ten days after this is done you will start feeling a little better and then gradually things will improve little by little. In two or three weeks the soreness will start going away."

"Will things ever be the same?"

"No, we did quite a lot of damage to get this right. Your taste may come back some, but not all the way back. You might always have some of the wattle that we gave you. You neck will always feel stiff from the surgeries. The radiation may degrade your hearing. Your teeth are going to be fragile without the saliva and because the radiation has changed the composition of your bones. Also the chemo may have messed with your kidneys. We'll see. So to answer your question - No, a few things will not be the same as they were but some things will come back a little, like your taste and your strength. Just keep hanging in there and do what you can."

"What's the best that can happen?"

He looked at me and thought for a second or two. "The best that can happen is that you are fine and I run into you about ten years from now in a department store. We say hello, we shake hands, you tell me you are living your life and that all is well. You tell me Susan and yourself are coming up on your next wedding anniversary and that all your children and grandchildren are doing fine. At that point I will know that I have done my job."

"That's good with me. I just want to tell you, thank you for everything you have done. Thank you for giving me a chance." My voice choked up.

"It's okay, that's what we do."

"No, you and Dr. Lee as well as everybody else have done everything they could to save me. Thanks for doing what you do. I don't know how you do it, but Thank You." I tear came down my cheek. "Thank you."

"You are welcome. I'll see you soon."

I stuck my hand out and we shook. With that, he turned and walked out the door.

"That's sounds good," Susan, who was with me for this, like every other appointment, said.

"Yep so far, so good. Now I just have to get through today and tomorrow and then start to recover. Did you buy any more protein drinks?"

"I did. I got some chocolate and some strawberry."

"Yesterday I tried the strawberry and I tasted it a little but the taste seemed off. It didn't taste right at all."

"Like Celeste said a few weeks ago, your taste may be altered by what you have gone through."

"I know. One more day and then hopefully we'll start to recover."

We stood up and walked out of the examining room and split up at the intersection of Waiting and Treatment.

And here I am, getting zapped for the penultimate time.

Fire away you metal and plastic mercenary. You get me for today and tomorrow and that's it.

After today and tomorrow either you will have done your work or you will not have done your work. Either way I can never be hooked up to you again. You gave me a lifetime dose in thirty-five days. Congratulations to you.

Here's to good shooting, Tex.

Day 35 – Tuesday - July 19, 2011

"Magnum PI Aloha Scrubs?" Mike was wearing red scrubs with huge Yellow Hibiscus and Bird of Paradise Flowers all over them.

"That's right Steve, I did it just for you."

"The top is fine but the bottom looks a little strange. But thank you, I think."

"It's hard to believe this is the last time I'll be bolting you in for liftoff. I'll be sad to see you go."

"No disrespect, but I won't be sad to go. I love you and all, but if I am never bolted into a machine like this again it will be too soon. I'll be sad to not see you as much, but I won't be sad about never coming into this room again. After today you can take my taped name off that locker over there. I hope that you never have to fill that locker up again with somebody else's form fitting contraption."

"We already have somebody to replace you."

"That sucks, it must be a never ending wheel for you. Do you ever feel like a hamster, spinning this damn thing round and round?"

"No. I do it because I'm good at it and I can help people. I do it because hopefully we save people's lives."

"Is it hard to do day after day?"

"Oh yeah, there are many times I feel like quitting. Sometimes no matter what we do this doesn't work and we lose people."

"So how do you do it then?"

"You just do it, hoping that you are doing more good than bad. Somebody has to do it. I can handle it for now. Hell I've been here for about ten years and have had about six or seven different partners helping me. Someday I'll burn out, but until then it's my job to keep going. Let's get you strapped in for the last time."

"Let's." I reclined and let Mike do his thing.

"See you later."

One thousand one, One thousand two, One thousand three, One thousand four…

I looked around me as much as I could. It was so different now, but so much the same. I no longer felt as much fear, but now I felt a strange mixture of gratitude and hate. I hated that this machine had ripped me up, but at the same time I was grateful that I lived in a time and place that I had a shot at making it. This machine didn't exist twenty years ago and hopefully it wouldn't need to exist twenty years from now.

:::::Wouldn't that be great.:::::

Yes, it would be great.

The machine started its warm up cycle and the lights started to flash. Soon the cylinder began to tumble around me and invisibly shoot through my skin and into my tissue and muscle under it, delicately destroying everything that it precisely touched. More damage, more damage and more damage, little by little, thirty-five days' worth.

This is your last shot at me, machine. Make it good. Eradicate all the bad stuff.

Please God, get rid of all the bad so this never comes back. Please.

I watched the lights go over. Only a couple more passes and we would be done. Get it good.

One thousand seven hundred and twenty-six, only one hundred and seventy-four more seconds to go.

Please God let everyone who figured this out and decided how much radiation I needed to get rid of this have gotten this right.

One thousand eight hundred and thirty-seven.

It slowly moved over once again. One more pass, one more pass over me, out of the hundreds and hundreds of passes it had made during the last month and a half.

One thousand eight hundred and sixty-two.

Was all my cancer gone now? Was this last pass or the chemo going to finish it off or would they not get everything. I guess those were the three alternatives. Please let it be one of the first two. Please.

Please save me. I have so much to live for.

Over it went for the last time.

One thousand nine hundred and four.

I started to cry.

It stopped above me and the lights began to flicker. Off they went, one by one. Through my tears I watched as the blurred last light slowly dimmed and then died.

One thousand nine-hundred and twenty-six.

Please, please, please let it all be gone. Please.

I was done with this damn machine. I loved it and I also hated it. I both loved it and hated it for making me evaluate myself. This thing tore me down both physically and mentally and hopefully now I could build myself back up again.

I heard Mike come into the room and saddle up beside me.

"Get this thing off of me."

"Hold on, I'm going as fast as I can."

He unscrewed the last fastener and lifted off my restraint. I quickly sat up, rubbed my eyes and deeply breathed in the medicinal air. I looked back at my captor. "Is that all you got?"

"Yep, that's it."

I didn't have the heart to tell Mike I wasn't talking to him. I stood up.

"Well?" Mike asked.

"Well what?"

He held up my restraint. “Do you want this? If you don’t take it, it’s going in the trash.”

I thought about it for less than a second. “Chuck it.”

“Good idea.” He put it down. “It goes in the trash soonest.”

We shook hands. “Thank you,” I said.

“Keep hanging in there.”

“Aloha.” I smiled and headed out of the chamber, down the hall and into the waiting room.

A couple of minutes later Susan and I headed up to the Chemo Room for the last time.

“Hold on,” I said before we started down the hallway into the room. The hallway looked a lot shorter now than it did six or seven weeks ago.

“What’s up?”

“Nothing. I don’t want to go in there again. I wish we could just turn around now. Why can’t it be done now?”

“Because it can’t. This is all you have left and then you can go home and rest for a month. No more doctors, no more coming here every day. Just rest and feel better and start doing things again. I love you.”

“I love you too. Thanks for getting me through this. Without you I would have turned and run away from this a hundred times.”

“I know.”

"I bet you do. Thanks for being with me every step. I'm sorry for all the times I have hurt you. I am so sorry for making you sick. I am…."

"Stop. Enough of that," she said.

We headed on in, I gave them my ID and we picked a spot for my treatment.

"Last one?" the nurse said as she brought over the magic poison.

"Yep, get it good."

She closed in on my arm and adeptly slid in the needle and hooked up the bags. Only four hours to go.

"You know the drill," she said. "Drink plenty of water and relax. You'll be done in a few hours."

"Thanks"

"I'm going to take a rest, you can go for a while if you want," I said to Susan.

"No, I'm good for now."

I closed my eyes. Thank you Lord. Please let me get through this and let me get better. Thank you for giving me all that you have given me. A loving wife, children, grandchildren. A career that made a difference.

:::::You have to do better.:::::

I do. I have to be a better husband, a better father, a better grandfather.

:::::You need to find something that will help others.:::::

I will.

:::::You need to help Stuart.:::::

I will. Thank you for the chance at helping my grandson. Maybe this can be the start of doing things better for me. I need to start working out of this funk. I've been given a second chance, at least for a while, and I need to take advantage of it.

"I AM ALWAYS WITH YOU."

My eyes opened and I looked around. Susan sat near me, taking in a *Reader's Digest.*

"Did you hear that?" I asked her.

"What?"

"Did somebody just say something?"

"Nobody said anything. Go back to resting."

I closed my eyes and shook it off.

"I AM ALWAYS WITH YOU."

I opened my eyes again and clearly nobody was around other than Susan and she didn't say anything.

"I AM ALWAYS WITH YOU." This time my eyes were open, but there was nobody around who could have said those words.

Where was it coming from? Who was it? It wasn't a normal voice in my head. This one was different, one I'd never heard before. I closed my eyes.

Who could it be? There were so many people with me. My mind and my soul were made up of so many different people. Weren't they all here with me right now, in this place, in some way?

My father, the man who raised me, the man to taught me so much while we fought most of our lives, he was here with me now.

My grandmother and my grandfather, those who took care of me before I was adopted, they molded me before they passed on and passed me on, they are here with me now.

Commander Gabovchik, he molded me into a Naval Officer, part of him is here with me now and always will be here with me.

All those I ever came in touch with, they are here with me now.

Every bad decision I ever made is here with me now. Every good decision I ever made is here with me now.

Everything I ever did is here with me now.

My wife, my children, my grandchildren, they are all here with me now.

Generation upon generation, five thousand of them. Every life has touched me somehow, fourteen billion of them. They have all made me what I am today, what I was in the past and what I may be in the future.

"I AM ALWAYS WITH YOU."

This voice was them, but it was not them. It was the voice that had pulled me through all this.

I am not crazy, I know I am not. This voice was partially my internal voices, it was partly the voices of all whom I have come in contact with, but it was more than that.

You decide what it was. I have decided that it's the voice of something higher than I, something greater than I.

It wasn't the voice that let me know that I would be okay. It was the voice that let me know it was always with me and that was enough. Good, bad or indifferent, it was always with me.

Somehow it brought me some peace after the past five terrifying months.

I turned to Susan, "I love you."

ABOUT THE AUTHOR

Stephen Krueger is the author of *Island of the Son* and *Ten Thousand and a Wake-Up*. He is a retired U.S. Navy Commander who began his career as a Seaman Recruit. After retiring from the Navy he earned his BA in English from the University of Hawai'i. He was born in Milwaukee and raised in Belize.

He is a cancer survivor.

www.ingramcontent.com/pod-product-compliance
Lightning Source LLC
Chambersburg PA
CBHW050109280326
41933CB00010B/1024
* 9 7 8 0 6 9 2 5 6 0 8 2 2 *